Faith in Older People

Registered Charity SC038225
Registered Company SC322915

21a Grosvenor Crescent
EDINBURGH EH12 5EL
Tel: 0131 346 7981

Email: info@fiop.org.uk
Website: fiop@dioceseofedinburgh.org

Elizabeth MacKinlay, RN, PhD
James W. Ellor, PhD, DMin, DCSW
Stephen Pickard, PhD
Editors

Aging, Spirituality and Pastoral Care: A Multi-National Perspective

Aging, Spirituality and Pastoral Care: A Multi-National Perspective has been co-published simultaneously as *Journal of Religious Gerontology*, Volume 12, Numbers 3/4 2001.

Pre-publication REVIEWS, COMMENTARIES, EVALUATIONS . . .

"This IMPRESSIVE, MULTIDISCIPLINARY COLLECTION OF SEMINAL ESSAYS on ethical and spiritual challenges in an aging society includes attention to topics such as late-life wisdom, integrity, spirituality, and sexuality. Even highly experienced pastors, counselors, geriatricians, and gerontologists will learn much from this stimulating book. IT DESERVES A PROMINENT PLACE AS A REQUIRED TEXTBOOK in theological schools and as enlightening supplemental reading to enrich human service scholars, scientists, and professionals."

David O. Moberg, PhD
Sociology Professor Emeritus
Marquette University
Milwaukee, Wisconsin

More Pre-publication
REVIEWS, COMMENTARIES, EVALUATIONS...

" **A** WEALTH OF MATERIAL....
Pastors, church leaders, and anyone concerned with what it means to grow older will find this book enlightening. The authors provide a valuable resource that engages and challenges the reader for ministry with older adults in the twenty-first century."

Rev. Richard H. Gentzler, Jr., DMin
Director, Center on Aging and Older Adult Ministries
The United Methodist Church
Nashville, Tennessee

" **C** OMPREHENSIVE....
The authors are not just thinkers and scholars. They speak from decades of practical expertise with the aged, demented, and dying."

Bishop Tom Frame, PhD
Lecturer in Public Theology
St. Mark's National Theological Centre
Canberra, Australia

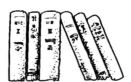

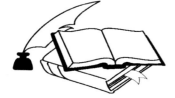

"The authors and editors have done a valuable service in bringing together scholarly and practical resources. . . . I WOULD NOT HESITATE TO USE IT AS A PRIMARY RESOURCE IN A SEMINARY COURSE ON AGING, nor to recommend it to colleagues in parish or institutional ministry with older persons. The chapter by Lamb and Thomson alone is worth the price of the book."

Rev. Robert W. Carlson, DMin
Chairman
The National Interfaith Coalition
on Aging
Chevy Chase Maryland
formerly Professor of Ministries
Seabury-Western Theological Seminary

The Haworth Pastoral Press
An Imprint of The Haworth Press, Inc.

Aging, Spirituality and Pastoral Care: A Multi-National Perspective

Aging, Spirituality and Pastoral Care: A Multi-National Perspective has been co-published simultaneously as *Journal of Religious Gerontology*, Volume 12, Numbers 3/4 2001.

The *Journal of Religious Gerontology* Monographic "Separates" (formerly Journal of Religion & Aging)*

Below is a list of " separates," which in serials librarianship means a special issue simultaneously published as a special journal issue or double-issue *and* as a "separate" hardbound monograph. (This is a format which we also call a "DocuSerial.")

"Separates" are published because specialized libraries or professionals may wish to purchase a specific thematic issue by itself in a format which can be separately cataloged and shelved, as opposed to purchasing the journal on an on-going basis. Faculty members may also more easily consider a "separate" for classroom adoption.

"Separates" are carefully classified separately with the major book jobbers so that the journal tie-in can be noted on new book order slips to avoid duplicate purchasing.

You may wish to visit Haworth's website at . . .

http://www.HaworthPress.com

. . . to search our online catalog for complete tables of contents of these separates and related publications.

You may also call 1-800-HAWORTH (outside US/Canada: 607-722-5857), or Fax 1-800-895-0582 (outside US/Canada: 607-771-0012), or e-mail at:

getinfo@haworthpressinc.com

Aging, Spirituality and Pastoral Care: A Multi-National Perspective, edited by Rev. Elizabeth MacKinlay, RN, PhD, Rev. James W. Ellor, PhD, DMin, DCSW, and Rev. Stephen Pickard, PhD (Vol. 12, No. 3/4, 2001). *"Comprehensive . . . The authors are not just thinkers and scholars. They speak from decades of practical expertise with the aged, demented, and dying." (Bishop Tom Frame, PhD, Lecturer in Public Theology, St. Mark's National Theological Centre, Canberra, Australia)*

Religion and Aging: An Anthology of the Poppele Papers, edited by Derrel R. Watkins, PhD, ACSW (Vol. 12, No. 2, 2001). *"Within these pages, the new ministry leader is supplied with the core prerequisites for effective older adult ministry and the more experienced leader is provided with an opportunity to reconnect with timeless foundational principles. Insights into the interior of the aging experience, field-tested and proven techniques and ministry principles, theological rationale for adult care giving, Biblical perspectives on aging, and philosophic and spiritual insights into the aging process." (Dennis R. Myers, LMSW-ACP, Director, Baccalaureate Studies in Social Work, Baylor University, Waco, Texas)*

Viktor Frankl's Contribution to Spirituality and Aging, edited by Melvin A. Kimble, PhD (Vol 11, No. 3/4, 2000). *Presents varying professional perspectives on the application of Frankl's logotherapy for ministry with older adults. Addresses issues such as death and dying, dementia and depression, and the spiritual meaning of aging.*

Aging in Chinese Society: A Holistic Approach to the Experience of Aging in Taiwan and Singapore, edited by Homer Jernigan and Margaret Jernigan (Vol. 8, No. 3, 1992). *"A vivid introduction to aging in these societies . . . Case studies illustrate the interaction of religion, personality, immigration, modernization, and aging." (Clinical Gerontologist)*

Spiritual Maturity in the Later Years, edited by James J. Seeber (Vol. 7, No. 1/2, 1991). *"An excellent introduction to the burgeoning field of gerontology and religion." (Southwestern Journal of Theology)*

Gerontology in Theological Education: Local Program Development, edited by Barbara Payne and Earl D. C. Brewer* (Vol. 6, No. 3/4, 1989). *"Directly relevant to gerontological education in other contexts and to applications in the educational programs and other work of church congregations and community agencies for the aging." (The Newsletter of the Christian Sociological Society)*

Gerontology in Theological Education, edited by Barbara Payne and Earl D. C. Brewer* (Vol. 6, No. 1/2, 1989) *"An excellent resource for seminaries and anyone interested in the role of the* *church in the lives of older persons. . . . must for all libraries."* (David Maldonado, DSW, Associate Professor of Church & Society, Southern Methodist University, Perkins School of Theology)

Religion, Aging and Health: A Global Perspective, compiled by the World Health Organization, edited by William M. Clements* (Vol. 4, No. 3/4, 1989) *"Fills a long-standing gap in gerontological literature. This book presents an overview of the interrelationship of religion, aging, and health from the perspective of the world's major faith traditions that is not available elsewhere . . . "* (Stephen Sapp, PhD, Associate Professor of Religious Studies, University of Miami, Coral Gables, Florida)

New Directions in Religion and Aging, edited by David B. Oliver* (Vol. 3, No. 1/2, 1987). *"This book is a telescope enabling us to see the future. The data of the present provides a solid foundation for seeing the future."* (Dr. Nathan Kollar, Professor of Religious Studies and Founding Chair, Department of Gerontology, St. John Fisher College; Adjunct Professor of Ministerial Theology, St. Bernard's Institute)

The Role of the Church in Aging, Volume 3: Programs and Services for Seniors, edited by Michael C. Hendrickson* (Vol. 2, No. 4, 1987). *"Experts explore an array of successful programs for the elderly that have been implemented throughout the United States in order to meet the social, emotional, religious, and health needs of the elderly."*

The Role of the Church in Aging, Volume 2: Implications for Practice and Service, edited by Michael C. Hendrickson* (Vol. 2, No. 3, 1986). *"Filled with important insight and state-of-the-art concepts that reflect the cutting edge of thinking among religion and aging professionals."* (Rev. James W. Ellor, DMin, AM, CSW, ACSW, Associate Professor, Department Chair, Human Service Department, National College of Education, Lombard, Illinois)

The Role of the Church in Aging, Volume 1: Implications for Policy and Action, edited by Michael C. Hendrickson* (Vol. 2, No. 1/2, 1986). *"Reviews the current status of the religious sector's involvement in the field of aging and identifies a series of strategic responses for future policy and action.*

Published by

The Haworth Pastoral Press, 10 Alice Street, Binghamton, NY 13904-1580 USA

The Haworth Pastoral Press is an imprint of The Haworth Press, Inc., 10 Alice Street, Binghamton, NY 13904-1580 USA.

Aging, Spirituality and Pastoral Care: A Multi-National Perspective has been co-published simultaneously as *Journal of Religious Gerontology*, Volume 12, Numbers 3/4 2001.

The development, preparation, and publication of this work has been undertaken with great care. However, the publisher, employees, editors, and agents of The Haworth Press and all imprints of The Haworth Press, Inc., including The Haworth Medical Press® and The Pharmaceutical Products Press®, are not responsible for any errors contained herein or for consequences that may ensue from use of materials or information contained in this work. Opinions expressed by the author(s) are not necessarily those of The Haworth Press, Inc.

Cover design by Thomas J. Mayshock Jr.

Library of Congress Cataloging-in-Publication Data

Aging, spirituality and pastoral care: a multi-national perspective / Elizabeth MacKinlay, James W. Ellor, and Stephen Pickard editors.
    p. cm.
  Includes bibliographical references and index.
  ISBN 0-7890-1668-0 (alk. paper) – ISBN 0-7890-1669-9 (pbk: alk. paper)
   1. Church work with the aged. 2. Aged–Religious life. I. MacKinlay, Elizabeth, 1940- II. Ellor, James W. III. Pickard, Stephen K.
BV4435 .A35 2002
259′.3–dc21
                                                  2002017168

Aging, Spirituality and Pastoral Care: A Multi-National Perspective

Elizabeth MacKinlay, RN, PhD
James W. Ellor, PhD, DMin, DCSW
Stephen Pickard, PhD
Editors

Aging, Spirituality and Pastoral Care: A Multi-National Perspective has been co-published simultaneously as *Journal of Religious Gerontology*, Volume 12, Numbers 3/4 2001.

The Haworth Pastoral Press
An Imprint of
The Haworth Press, Inc.
New York • London • Oxford

Indexing, Abstracting & Website/Internet Coverage

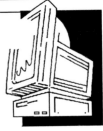

This section provides you with a list of major indexing & abstracting services. That is to say, each service began covering this periodical during the year noted in the right column. Most Websites which are listed below have indicated that they will either post, disseminate, compile, archive, cite or alert their own Website users with research-based content from this work. (This list is as current as the copyright date of this publication.)

Abstracting, Website/Indexing Coverage . . . . Year When Coverage Began

- *Abstracts in Social Gerontology: Current Literature on Aging* **1991**

- *AgeInfo CD-ROM* **1994**

- *AgeLine Database* **1994**

- *Applied Social Sciences Index & Abstracts (ASSIA) (Online: ASSI via Data-Star) (CD-Rom: ASSIA Plus) <http://www.bowker-saur.co.uk>* **1994**

- *BUBL Information Service, an Internet-based Information Service for the UK higher education community <URL: http://bubl.ac.uk/>* **1999**

- *CNPIEC Reference Guide: Chinese National Directory of Foreign Periodicals* **1995**

- *Educational Administration Abstracts (EAA)* **1995**

- *Family & Society Studies Worldwide <www.nisc.com>* **1996**

- *FINDEX <www.publist.com>* **1999**

- *Guide to Social Science & Religion in Periodical Literature* **2000**

(continued)

Special Bibliographic Notes related to special journal issues (separates) and indexing/abstracting:

- indexing/abstracting services in this list will also cover material in any "separate" that is co-published simultaneously with Haworth's special thematic journal issue or DocuSerial. Indexing/abstracting usually covers material at the article/chapter level.
- monographic co-editions are intended for either non-subscribers or libraries which intend to purchase a second copy for their circulating collections.
- monographic co-editions are reported to all jobbers/wholesalers/approval plans. The source journal is listed as the "series" to assist the prevention of duplicate purchasing in the same manner utilized for books-in-series.
- to facilitate user/access services all indexing/abstracting services are encouraged to utilize the co-indexing entry note indicated at the bottom of the first page of each article/chapter/contribution.
- this is intended to assist a library user of any reference tool (whether print, electronic, online, or CD-ROM) to locate the monographic version if the library has purchased this version but not a subscription to the source journal.
- individual articles/chapters in any Haworth publication are also available through the Haworth Document Delivery Service (HDDS).

Aging, Spirituality and Pastoral Care: A Multi-National Perspective

CONTENTS

SECTION 2: ISSUES OF AGEING AND PASTORAL CARE

ABOUT THE EDITORS

Elizabeth MacKinlay, RN, PhD, is a Registered Nurse and priest in the Anglican Church of Australia. She has focused on care of the aging since the early 1980s. She wrote her dissertation on the spiritual dimension of aging in independent-living older people. Since then she has undertaken further research with frail older residents of nursing homes and people living with dementia. She is currently a senior lecturer at University of Canberra and Director of the Centre for Ageing and Pastoral Studies. She is also a sessional lecturer at the Charles Sturt University School of Theology.

James W. Ellor, PhD, DMin, DCSW, is a social worker and an ordained Presbyterian minister. He is Professor of Human Services and Gerontology at National-Louis University, where he has worked for more than 18 years. He is also Associate Director of the Center for Aging, Religion and Spirituality; Interim Director of Pastoral Care at Westminster Presbyterian Church in Aurora, Illinois; and an on-call chaplain at Edward Hospital. He is the senior editor of the *Journal of Religious Gerontology* and editor-in-chief of The Haworth Pastoral Press. He has written and lectured widely in this field.

Stephen Pickard, PhD, is Associate Professor and Head of the School of Theology at Charles Sturt University. The university is in partnership with St. Mark's National Theological Centre, Canberra, where Stephen is Director. He has been an Anglican priest for twenty years, during which time he has served in parish and chaplaincy work in Australia and the United Kingdom. His area of professional interest is in theology, church, and society.

Preface

The idea for this double volume grew out of the preparations for the first international conference, *Ageing, Spirituality and Pastoral Care in the Twenty-First Century* held in Canberra, Australia in January 2000. As people accepted invitations to speak at the conference it became evident that there was developing a critical body of knowledge that would be presented at this conference. The main invited speakers came from a range of disciplines of gerontology, bringing with them a richness of worldviews of what it means to be growing older at the beginning of the twenty-first century.

The chapters produced in this volume cover a range of material that we have endeavoured to group, both sequentially as the papers were presented at the conference, and by theme as a progression, beginning with ethical issues emerging for ageing societies.

Dr. Laurie McNamara has drawn an ethical map that lays a basis for considering quality of life issues in ageing for individuals and the wider community. Professor Mel Kimble has engaged with issues of meaning in later life, moving beyond the biomedical paradigm. Professor John Painter has written on the biblical picture of ageing. Following these three chapters that set the scene and tone for the rest of the chapters, a jointly written chapter by Dr. Winifred Lamb and Heather Thomson considers the ageing self. This chapter focuses on the philosophical and theological aspects of the ageing self. Professor Don Thomson's chapter takes yet another perspective of ageing, that of wisdom and the ageing process. These five chapters complete this initial section.

The next section considers issues of ageing. First is Elizabeth MacKinlay's outline of social and spiritual isolation in ageing, and the need for intimacy for older people. Dr. Jim Seeber's chapter looks at a theological perspective . . . Dr. Elizabeth MacKinlay's outline of social

---

[Haworth co-indexing entry note]: "Preface." MacKinlay, Elizabeth. Co-published simultaneously in *Journal of Religious Gerontology* (The Haworth Pastoral Press, an imprint of The Haworth Press, Inc.) Vol. 12, No. 3/4, 2001, pp. xxi-xxii; and: *Aging, Spirituality and Pastoral Care: A Multi-National Perspective* (ed: Elizabeth MacKinlay, James W. Ellor, and Stephen Pickard) The Haworth Pastoral Press, an imprint of The Haworth Press, Inc., 2001, pp. xiii-xiv. Single or multiple copies of this article are available for a fee from The Haworth Document Delivery Service [1-800-342-9678, 9:00 a.m. - 5:00 p.m. (EST). E-mail address: getinfo@haworth pressinc.com].

xiii

and spiritual isolation in ageing, and the need for intimacy for older people on sexuality and ageing. This chapter looks at a theological perspective of sexuality and pastoral responses that consider older peoples' attitudes towards sexual relationships in later life. The topic of spiritual and psychological development in later life is considered in the context of a study of knowledge of the spiritual dimension and raising that awareness amongst a group of nurses working in six different nursing homes. This chapter is written by Dr. MacKinlay.

The following section contains topics of a more practical focus. Rev. Malcolm Goldsmith's contribution is of two chapters that address particular issues of living with dementia and connecting with people who have dementia. Dr. Elizabeth MacKinlay's article examines the spiritual dimension of caring, while Dr. Anne van Loon describes a model for parish nursing practice.

Finally, a homily preached at an ecumenical service during the conference by Professor Stephen Pickard is included as an epilogue, challenging attitudes towards ageing.

Rev. Elizabeth MacKinlay, RN, PhD
Senior Lecturer
University of Canberra
Canberra, ACT
Australia

Director of the Centre for Aging and Pastoral Studies
St. Marks National Theological Centre
Canberra, ACT
Australia

Honorary Assistant Priest
Anglican Church of the Good Shepherd
Canberra, ACT
Australia

Introduction

Frequently, persons working in the area of Spiritual and Religious concerns of older adults feel very alone, whether he or she is involved in ministry, social service, nursing or other human service tasks. In this volume, authors from Australia, England, and the United States come together to offer their insights and perspectives on our common journey with seniors. As I have the opportunity to talk with colleagues from all over the world, I am impressed with the common struggles that we all have. How do I integrate my three worlds, my professional orientation, my understanding of the aging process, and my knowledge of the spiritual needs of seniors? The authors in this volume draw together their voices to respond to these concerns.

Particularly colleagues in our common ministry in Australia and the United States have more in common that many may recognize. Our two countries have our common roots in the British Empire, European Christian Theologies and culture as well as many socio-economic realities. There are also some differences. When Dr. MacKinlay and I put the following thoughts together the first thing we found was that statistics are often not calculated the same in the two countries. However, many of the trends are very much the same. Indeed, the richness of our diversity clearly finds resonance in all that we have in common.

AUSTRALIA AND THE UNITED STATES, PARTNERS IN SPIRITUAL PATHS IN AGING

Mrs. Smith is 97 years old. She and her husband have raised two daughters after her husband came back from Europe from the first

[Haworth co-indexing entry note]: "Introduction." Ellor, James W. Co-published simultaneously in *Journal of Religious Gerontology* (The Haworth Pastoral Press, an imprint of The Haworth Press, Inc.) Vol. 12, No. 3/4, 2001, pp. 1-4; and: *Aging, Spirituality and Pastoral Care: A Multi-National Perspective* (ed: Elizabeth MacKinlay, James W. Ellor, and Stephen Pickard) The Haworth Pastoral Press, an imprint of The Haworth Press, Inc., 2001, pp. 1-4. Single or multiple copies of this article are available for a fee from The Haworth Document Delivery Service [1-800-342-9678, 9:00 a.m. - 5:00 p.m. (EST). E-mail address: getinfo@haworthpressinc.com].

war to end all wars. Her husband died nineteen years ago. She lives alone in an assisted living facility that costs $800 dollars a month. She has Medicare, Social Security and a small pension from her work as an elementary school teacher. She is a member of St. Mary's Roman Catholic Church, but she is generally unable to attend, as she does not get out much. A woman from the church, who also brings communion, visits her from time to time.

Mr. Taylor is 81 years old. He went into the Navy right after college to fight in World War II. After the war, he married his High School Sweetheart. Together they raised one son and a daughter. His son fought in Vietnam and was killed. He and his wife have been members of Our Savior Baptist Church since they were married. They now live in a nursing home that was built by their church as Mrs. Taylor has dementia and needs a great deal of care. They have Medicare for some assistance, but mostly rely on his pension and their Social Security. Their church continues to be very important, both to support him through the trials of his wife's condition as well as to offer spiritual support to her as she has slowly lost the ability to remember his name. He particularly finds reading scripture to be helpful in times of stress.

What country do Mr. Taylor or Mrs. Smith live in, Australia, or the United States? The answer is, that from these descriptions they could live in either country. While Australia and the United States each have their own distinct histories and important stories to tell, the similarities and common concerns are overwhelming. Both countries began as colonies of England. Both countries were settled in part by the criminals and debtors sent from England to Georgia in the United States and to New South Wales and Tasmania in Australia. Both countries had wilderness areas to concur, and unfortunately, both countries tried to eliminate the indigenous communities of people who lived there prior to the landing of Europeans. Both countries fought in the two world wars as well as in Vietnam.

As both countries' majority populations emigrated from Europe, their religious histories are also intertwined. Both have strong Roman Catholic, as well as Protestant populations. When talking about the influence of the Protestant Reformation, both turn to the work of Martin Luther and John Calvin. Dialogue between clergy and laypersons from these two countries suggest that spiritual issues are very much the same in these two countries.

The landmass of Australia and the lower 48 states of the United States is similar. However, Australia has fewer total persons. Even so, the population patterns are similar. In both countries the impact of the "baby boom" "reaching 'golden pond,' " will have the effect of greatly exploding the number of persons who are older, on pensions and in need of long term care. As seen in Table 1, the percentages of persons growing old as well as the lower percentage of persons in the work force are similar.

One can see from both the historic and demographic data that families in both the United States and Australia struggle with very similar demographic, emotional, physical health and spiritual issues. This

TABLE 1. Comparison of Demographic Data Between Australia and the United States[1]

Topic	United States	Australia
Year baby boom reaches 65	2011	2011
Percent persons over 65 in year 2030	20%	
There are more older women than men	True	True
The proportion of older adults to total population varies by state	True	True
More older men than women are currently married	True	True
Percent of persons living in poverty	11%	
Life Expectancy	77.1	79.8
Percent of persons 65+ who suffer from some type of memory loss	4%	5% Direct Comparisons can not be accurately calculated
Percent who live in Nursing Homes Age 65-74 Age 85 + (Source: U.S. Census Bureau Statistical Brief 1995)	1% 25%	2.4% (these figures are for all aged care institutions) 39.2%, i.e., hostels and nursing homes ABS 1999

[1] 2000. Older Americans 2000: Key Indicators of Well-Being. Washington DC: Federal Interagency Forum on Aging and Related Statistics.

would suggest that each country has a lot to learn by working with scholars and pastors from the other. In this volume, authors from Australia, the United States and Great Britain have come together to offer their insights into the spiritual needs of older adults.

Rev. James W. Ellor, PhD, DMin, DCSW,
ACSW, BCD, DCSW, CGP
Editor
Journal of Religious Gerontology

Professor
National-Louis University
200 South Naperville Road
Wheaton, Illinois 60187 USA

Associate Director
Center for Aging, Religion and Spirituality
St. Paul, Minnesota USA

Interim Director of Pastoral Care
Westminster Presbyterian Church
Aurora, Illinois USA

Rev. Elizabeth MacKinlay, RN, PhD
Senior Lecturer
University of Canberra
Canberra, ACT
Australia

Director of the Centre for Aging and Pastoral Studies
St. Marks National Theological Centre
Canberra, ACT
Australia

Honorary Assistant Priest
Anglican Church of the Good Shepherd
Canberra, ACT
Australia

SECTION 1:
ETHICAL, THEOLOGICAL
AND BIBLICAL DIMENSIONS

Ethics and Ageing in the 21st Century

Laurence J. McNamara, CM, PhD

SUMMARY. This article insists that a cautious view of population data about ageing is necessary. Against this background three questions of meaning are explored, namely, what does it mean to grow old? What does it mean to be healthy or ill when one is old? What does it mean to care for aged persons in an age of chronic illness and disability? These questions raise justice issues about distribution of resources and quality of life and bring into focus theological insights about the human person, human solidarity and human virtues in a way that contributes to public discourse about ethics and ageing. *[Article copies available for a fee from The Haworth Document Delivery Service: 1-800-342-9678. E-mail address: <getinfo@haworthpressinc.com> Website: <http://www.HaworthPress.com> © 2001 by The Haworth Press, Inc. All rights reserved.]*

Dr. Laurence J. McNamara, is a Catholic Priest of the Congregation of the Mission (Vincentians) and Senior Lecturer in Christian Ethics and Deputy-President of The Catholic Institute of Sydney.

Address correspondence to: Dr. Laurence J. McNamara, Catholic Institute of Sydney, 99 Albert Road, Sydney NSW 2135, Australia (E-mail: lmcnamara@cis.catholic.edu.au).

[Haworth co-indexing entry note]: "Ethics and Ageing in the 21st Century." McNamara, Laurence J. Co-published simultaneously in *Journal of Religious Gerontology* (The Haworth Pastoral Press, an imprint of The Haworth Press, Inc.) Vol. 12, No. 3/4, 2001, pp. 5-29; and: *Aging, Spirituality and Pastoral Care: A Multi-National Perspective* (ed: Elizabeth MacKinlay, James W. Ellor, and Stephen Pickard) The Haworth Pastoral Press, an imprint of The Haworth Press, Inc., 2001, pp. 5-29. Single or multiple copies of this article are available for a fee from The Haworth Document Delivery Service [1-800-342-9678, 9:00 a.m. - 5:00 p.m. (EST). E-mail address: getinfo@haworthpressinc.com].

5

KEYWORDS. Ageing, ethics, meaning, justice, quality-of-life, person, solidarity, virtue

INTRODUCTION

Over the last one hundred years the journey of life has extended significantly for an increasing proportion of our Australian population. The experience of increasing longevity brings with it important human questions of meaning, together with questions about the justice and quality of life to be expected as we age. These three issues constitute the central part of this paper. To appreciate their importance it will be necessary to introduce, if only briefly, relevant demographic factors and ethical considerations that influence any response that might be made to the matters in question. By way of conclusion three sets of values grounded in Christian theology will be discussed for they contribute in significant ways to ethical reflection on issues arising from human ageing and the ageing of our society.

DEMOGRAPHY AND ETHICS

The Population Question

Many who think about the 21st Century portray the greying of the population as one of the major global hazards to confront humanity. The combination of greater longevity and lower birthrates will trigger a crisis, they claim, that will engulf the world. During the next decade a trickle of "baby boomers" will be heading into retirement but by 2015 they will become a flood.[1] This scenario appears in newspapers and magazines frequently in reference to difficulties associated with allocating resources be they health care, housing, pensions or community care.

Those who resist this bleak view of the future argue that we should look beyond mere statistics. They point to the three underlying factors that influence the proportion of older people in society–namely birth, death and immigration rates. For many in Australia today much greater concern is expressed about the possible economic consequences for workers and tax payers that will result from an increasing proportion of ageing persons. This relationship between productive and non-productive sectors in the population (the so called *dependency ratio*) must be viewed with caution. It may be portrayed in terms of age alone, on the basis of those of working age (viz. 15-64 years), or more accurately in relation to labour force figures. When the latter perspective is taken current concerns have no basis.[2] Equally important, however, is the fact that private expenditure on dependent groups is much higher for children than for the elderly in our society. Parents provide the greater part of support to children whereas government expenditure dominates in the case of aged persons. In spite of this some have concluded from available data that the dependency ratio will increase at a slow rate in the coming decades.[3] Demographic data also indicate that throughout the early years of the 21st century Australia will continue to have a large proportion of the population of workforce age and relatively small groups in the categories of young and old. Australia's high birth and immigration rates of the post-World War II years will produce larger numbers of people who are retirees in 2011. This group will have entered the 'old' old group (80 years and above) by 2031.[4]

In light of this demographic profile it is possible to indicate a number of implications for ageing Australia. First, the nation is not experiencing nor will it experience acute population ageing, at least by world standards. This realisation should ground any ethical analysis. Secondly, during the next decade elderly persons from non-English speaking countries, many of whom came to Australia in the 1940s and 1950s, will be entering old-old age. This will necessitate the provision of culturally appropriate health, community and aged care services. Thirdly, indigenous Australians (Aborigines and Torres Strait Islanders) have not shared the increasing longevity of other Australians throughout the 20th century. High mortality among the young and middle-aged has resulted in a diminished proportion of indigenous people among our ageing population. Fourthly, social, economic and political factors must be included with any consideration of demographic factors associated with the ageing of the Australian population. Financing retirement and old age, housing, urban planning, transport and local amenities, health care and community services will have to be given increasing importance in any analysis of ageing in the 21st century. To think comprehensively in this manner confronts the prevailing economic rationalism dominating current public policy. Finally, ageing people are immersed in a world of rapid change. Because of this elderly Australians are not quarantined from the "crosscurrents, contradictions, uncertainties, ambiguities and paradoxes that characterise Australian attitudes at the end of the 20th century."[5] The task ahead for all Australians is to develop metaphors and patterns of meaning for the experiences of ageing in a fast changing world.

The Ethical Landscape

Three aspects of our cultural milieu significantly influence current discussions of ageing: postmodernity, pluralism and secularity. Hugh Mackay puts it well when he writes that

> Australia is becoming a truly postmodern society–a place where we are learning to incorporate uncertainty in our view of the world. The absolute is giving way to the relative; objectivity to subjectivity; function to form. In the modern view of the 20th century, seeing was believing; in the postmodern world of the turn of the century, believing is seeing. Conviction yields to speculation; prejudice to a new open-mindedness; religious dogma to a more intuitive, inclusive spirituality. Even the concept of God receives a changed emphasis, from the materialist's 'out-there' being, to a spirit that is more intimately part of us.[6]

In ethical terms there is a "loss of singular certainty about truth and right in contemporary societies."[7] The narrow utilitarian calculus of the modern era has the effect of creating winners and losers. Frequently the elderly, women and indigenous peoples are to be found among the latter group. It is the strength of postmodern thinking that the stance of particular individuals or groups is given priority. This accompanies a critical attitude to relationships of power and oppression. A post-modern focus has implications for current thinking on the role of ageing persons in society. Increasingly the place of the spirit and spirituality are being recognised in a way not possible within a scientific paradigm. As will be observed later in this paper this is particularly significant for any consideration of the experience of growing old in contemporary society.

In liberal societies such as our own substantive moral agreement is not required beyond the need for all to agree about mutual toleration of diversity. Pluralism acknowledges there is no one set of moral values and practices acceptable to all members of society such that they might be given the force of law.[8] A pluralist society rejects all views contrary to its own where individual freedom and mutual tolerance are concerned for these are foundational values in the liberal *polis*. Here the law is viewed as expressing a social consensus that individual freedom and mutual tolerance form the best basis for a society where many different worldviews and lifestyles exist.[9] One reaction to this state of affairs maintains that the truth of the post-modern condition is such that everyone must live with fragmentation and pluralism because reason cannot establish for *moral strangers* a concrete, content-full common vision of the moral life.[10]

Two observations are appropriate here. First, a pluralism grounded in notions of liberty and tolerance which sees individuals as moral strangers gives central importance to human autonomy and its corresponding ethic of choice. An ethos of freedom-through-choice and a correlative emphasis on the role of contracts in the ordering of social relations is, at times, at odds with the Christian emphasis on enduring commitments and fidelity. The latter are best characterised by the biblical notion of covenant. Second, a contractual framework of social relations gives priority to equality, impartiality and universality in human relations. As a consequence of this little or no consideration has been given in Anglo-American philosophy to the qualities present in emotional, familial and other relations of friendship. These manifest personal responsiveness and partiality where personal emotions and virtues enable the individual to discern and respond to the needs of others.

The third aspect of our current ethical landscape arises from the secularity of the developed world. From the beginnings of revelation two trajectories may be observed in humanity's dealings with God. One diminishes the influence of myth, fate or spiritual intermediaries as causes of human events and places at centre stage human responsibility for conduct. This secularisation of human morality is well illustrated in the first three chapters of the book of Genesis. The second trajectory maps the Old Testament struggle for faith in the one God who is holy and completely other. [11] In the Word made Flesh this God has "made his dwelling among us." [12]

Much has been written about the process of secularisation during the 20th century. A persuasive argument has been made that we should no longer view ourselves at the beginning of the 21st century as living in a secular *society*. Rather we should understand ourselves as immersed in a secular *culture*. Secular culture is not overtly hostile to faith; rather, it radically undermines it. Our commodified culture assumes we live for pleasure without commitment.[13] From the religious point of view secular culture has its greatest impact in the areas of imagination, disposition and sensibility. In place of old-style atheism with its militant and angry rejections the battle ground has moved deeper–into what Newman would call antecedent assumptions, those attitudinal preambles that either make faith existentially credible or incredible. If culture is in part a shared 'structure of feeling,' which silently shapes the images we live by, then a dominantly secular culture can quietly marginalize those ways of feeling-towards-God without which faith remains unborn or unreal. Moreover, in so far as the Churches remain within a complacently sacral language, they ignore that their own cultural and spiritual incredibility may be on a 'pre-religious' level. [14]

As a consequence a secular environment eclipses any sense of need or desire for anything more than immediacy.

Christian faith becomes not so much incredible as unimagined and even unimaginable. This is no longer a merely social or external phenomenon. It involves the secularization of the shared consciousness at the root of culture.[15]

This loss of both a sense of and sensitivity to the transcendent with its myths and symbols is being eroded by the world of the immediate with its market-driven values. This process of commodification of much in our modern world gives priority to efficiency, productivity and competitiveness reign. It trumpets an *ethic of achievement* that starkly contradicts the Christian theology and *ethic of being*. This dichotomy manifests itself most acutely in the lives of ageing persons. No longer productive in economic terms their contributions to social life simply by being elderly members of the community are hardly, if at all, valued.

The implications of demographic change and the reality of our ethical landscape provide the backdrop for the inquiry that follows. In the section that follows attention will be focused on three sets of questions that concern human ageing, namely questions of meaning, questions about justice and quality of life.

QUESTIONS

Questions of Meaning

The fundamental challenge confronting 21st century Australian society as it considers the ageing of its members is to address the question of meaning: "What does it mean to grow old?" Closely aligned with this question are two further questions that have particular importance as a greater proportion of the population lives into old age. First, "What does it mean to be healthy or ill when one is old?" and second, "What does it mean to care especially when elderly and frail people have chronic illness and disabilities?" It is to these three questions I now turn.

What Does It Mean to Grow Old?

The experience of ageing in the developed countries of the West occurs in societies permeated with a fear of death. Social attitudes view ageing as a period of non-productivity. The priority given to all things technical considers ageing as a pathology, the incurable disease of living. Growth and development, the dominant paradigm of life in the contemporary world, are portrayed primarily in terms of an increasing independence. Ageing, on the other hand, is viewed as decline, a downward spiral into dependency. In truth, however, real growth and development occur in an ever expanding network of obligations and dependencies throughout the entire journey of life. Being old is but one of a number of stages in life where each individual moves through one system of dependency to another.[16]

An understanding of ageing first emerges in the life of each person as a temporal concept, as a transition from one's past through the present toward the future.[17] As we grow older some parts of our bodies become rigid and others flaccid. Perhaps the hardening is a final structuring, a settling on what one's character and essence are to be, once and for all. The softening entails a dropping away of what one decides is not to be incorporated into the essential structure, the completed character. This does not mean that ageing is not a time of growth. It is a growing clearer and more decided about the essence, the form, that one wants one's existence to have, a growing firmer in those features that will be the defining shape of the person. At another level the experience of ageing comes with the experience of slowing down. Associated with this is a different sense of time. Ageing is that part of our lives where our being slows at all levels enabling the individual to experience situations and persons with more attentiveness and care. Many elderly persons come to realise that time has both a dimension of depth as well as duration. Ageing persons slow themselves to explore experiences, not in their linear pattern of succeeding one another, but in their possibility of opening for them entire worlds in each situation and in each person encountered. The ageing person comes to be more gentle with these experiences, to take care to let their possibilities and rich density emerge. The elderly continue moving through time, but they also move into time, allowing it to expand in depth even though its objective duration diminishes.

As one ages skin wrinkles and roughens, posture becomes curved. Memory is restructured. Formerly unbroken stretches of clarity are marked by peaks and between them hollows called confusion. Among all the changes and indicators of ageing, ambiguous as they are to the consciousness of the ageing person, death is foreseen. One more meaning of ageing that is recognised experientially, whether consciously or not, is that life is finite. The sum of all these changes in the experience of ageing persons indicates a tacit, organic knowledge that death is a reality, that *my* death is not something speculative but a *felt* reality in the very fabric of *my* existence.

The experience of increasing frailty is often delineated as a characteristic of ageing and old age. As a phenomenon it is intrinsic to all human experience. The frailty of older persons is, therefore, not a feature setting them apart from younger persons. Rather, an "unalterable given in human existence is the possibility of injury and destruction, the quality of frailty."[18] The meaning that is given to the experience of human frailty reflects the more general values our culture gives to its understanding of the human condition.

The ambiguity of one's subjective experience of ageing, the changing sense of time that comes with slowing down, the changes in the ageing person's physical body and the very profound sense of personal frailty are but some of the ways in which all who share the common human experience of ageing encounter the reality of longevity. As is obvious already the human mind seeks to grasp the experience, to understand it in some way.

At its core ageing is fundamentally a *mystery* rather than a *problem*. Failure to appreciate that ageing shares the dimension of mystery with life as a whole takes human inquiries into meaning along unsatisfactory paths. The ambiguities present in ageing frequently result in a tension between public and private understandings of what it means to grow old.[19] Scientific meanings of ageing are separated from and frequently have priority over experiential or existential understandings. This has implications for dealings with ageing persons. Not to prize their experience and how they have come to understand and give meaning to this part of their life journey has the effect of radically undermining their uniqueness, individuality and dignity. The philosophy, literature and arts of Western civilisation offer rich resources for building a broad humanistic understanding of the meaning of growing old. While it is not possible to open up this area in a short paper such as this, it is helpful to note, however, that our civic effort to explore the meaning of ageing and old age would be greatly enriched by using such resources.

Because much contemporary thinking is postmodern, pluralist and secular it fails in its attempt to answer the question as to what ageing means. I believe the Christian community has a theological understanding of ageing that situates more satisfactorily within its wider theological insights about *human life* and *death*. By framing ageing and old age within a theological understanding of human life and death we are able to transform the meaning of ageing and old age in a way that merely humanistic reflection or philosophical analysis are unable to achieve. A more adequate appreciation of the meaning of human ageing is to be found in a total life-span view that values life and death. Roman Catholic moral thinking views each person as having responsibility for living fully at every stage of life such that each phase directly prepares for the stages that follow. Ultimately life is a preparation for final union with God. Practical consequences flow from this total life-span view. One is that any social segmentation that isolates a group within the total community has a deleterious effect on the entire community. Where this occurs old age is devalued. Younger generations are at the same time effectively deprived of seeing their present life as directly linked to and preparatory for their later years. For aged persons themselves there is also the loss of those benefits that come with multi-generational living within the wider community.

What Does It Mean to Be Healthy or Ill When One Is an Aged Person?

Healthy people usually take their health for granted for to be healthy is to be freed from some of the limitations and problems that cause them to be self-reflective. It is not necessary to pause before getting up out of the chair, before walking to the door or doing odd jobs around the house. A state of bodily and psychic health remains as the background to healthy activity.[20] Illness, on the other hand, teaches humans the precariousness of this world. When illness comes a lack of health becomes evident. Many of the features of health which until now had been taken for granted are reflected on and recalled.

A number of things flow from this. First, an individual's relationship with his or her body must frequently be mediated through others, such as when the doctor makes a diagnosis or a nurse offers care. Second, the bodily dis-integration typical of illness suffuses the patient's experience of space and time. Confined to bed the sick person finds the way to the future blocked. Third, dis-unity with others frequently accompanies the dis-integration of illness. No longer part of the mainstream the sick person may feel at a distance from those who are healthy and who go about their daily lives. Loneliness can contribute greatly to the suffering of the ill. Fourth, the experience of illness raises deeper questions which cause the sick person to confront themselves and their place in the world. Because of the multi-dimensional character of illness the existence of the sick person is altered in a significant way.[21]

For the Christian human well-being is not a matter of holding on to health at any cost. Rather, true well-being involves both health and illness. Christian theology brackets its view of human well-being between notions of *human bodiliness* on the one hand and *pain and suffering* on the other. In a society deeply attached to bodily beauty and the capacity to function effectively, human bodiliness is frequently viewed as an instrumental value. A theological perspective, however, recognises that an ageing person's body is the privileged *locus* of care and attention. This is recognised no matter how limited, handicapped, disfigured or decrepit a particular person's body may be. In Roman Catholic thinking the body of the elderly person is sacramental, open to revealing mystery, especially the mystery of God.

Two of the most powerful dis-integrating forces in illness are the experience of pain and suffering. Pain asserts itself not only at the sensory level. It is also experienced spatially as either the contraction of the universe down to the immediate vicinity of the body or as the body swelling to fill the entire universe.[22] Pain influences, restructures and even dictates the sufferer's perceptions of time as is shown by the use of the words *chronic* and *chronology, endurance* and *duration*.[23] Pain also configures the body as something alien. Patients often describe their pain as an *it* separate from the *I*. The painful body is often experienced as something foreign to the self. In a society where secularism, hedonism and materialism are relatively powerful ideologies the reality of pain and suffering in human lives is a great conundrum. Many today deny that pain and suffering are inevitable. They reject any positive interpretation of this most difficult of human experiences. What results is the imposition of a rather odd and oppressive judgment on the sufferer for suffering is judged at times to be avoidable, at other times to be the result of a defective personality structure or due to a lack of enlightenment and even the consequence of irresponsible behaviour.

> If pain and suffering are not understood as part of our human lot but are approached as a correctable dysfunction, then the tragic dimension of human experience undergoes a radical change of status. The sufferer is blamed.[24]

The meaning of human pain and suffering has challenged human minds from the beginning of time. The Christian who searches for an answer to such questions is confronted by a God who is both radically holy and incomprehensibly mysterious. Acceptance of suffering thus becomes a significant faith event, an experience of trusting in the mysteriousness of the God whom we, like Job in the Old Testament, can never fully understand.[25] The link between faith and suffering is proclaimed most dramatically in the Church's major liturgical season of Lent as it reflects on the sufferings of the Saviour. In all of this the Christian is not glorifying suffering. Rather suffering is understood primarily in theological terms.[26]

The Bible takes suffering seriously. It does not minimise it, shows profound compassion for the sufferer and sees suffering as an evil which ought not to be.[27] Jesus, the man of sorrows, showed himself sensitive to all human suffering.[28] As the Christian now lives in Christ so the sufferings of the Christian are the sufferings of Christ in the believer.[29] If the believer suffers it is in order to be glorified with Christ.[30] For the Christian this is a privilege.[31] It merits eternal glory after death but also brings joy in this life.[32] There is joy for Paul in the sufferings he endured for he is able to "fill up in his flesh what is wanting to the sufferings of Christ for his body which is the church."[33] Throughout the biblical material the experience of pain and suffering takes on a cosmic dimension far different to contemporary philosophy with its individualistic and psychological preoccupations.[34]

Pain and suffering attack the integrity of human beings, not only those who suffer but also those who accompany the suffering person in their trial.[35] The person who suffers often experiences a sense of abandonment. People frequently turn from them leaving them isolated and alone in their anguish. Suffering involves all dimensions of human life: It speaks in physical pain, wreaks havoc in the soul and impairs human relationships. Although the Christian tradition cannot offer a ready explanation or a simple solution to the problem of suffering, it can nevertheless offer support in suffering and some guidance as to how one might respond to it.

Any approach to health and illness, pain and suffering in the lives of ageing persons must incorporate its spiritual dimension. Where a rich understanding of human bodiliness and the reality of pain and suffering are present it will be possible to elaborate a more comprehensive, and ultimately a more satisfying understanding of human well-being for all phases of the human life-span, especially old age.

What Does It Mean to Care When One Is Growing Old or Aged?

Caring is grounded in the vulnerability of the other. In situations of vulnerability the carer is required to accompany the patient in his or her experience of pain, loneliness and isolation. One of the most basic loyalties owed to another is the loyalty of watching, waiting, keeping company, standing by, and giving care to the sick, the dying and those in pain.[36] Not only is care expressed in words, it is also conveyed by sight and touch. Touch is a more compelling form of contact than either sight or hearing because it is the symbol of vulnerability. In the caring relationship the body is regarded and touched by the carer as the immediate lived reality of the other. Empathetic touch affirms, rather than ignores, the subjective significance of the body for the ageing person. Its purpose is to express the carer's participation in the aged person's experience. The caring relationship not only overcomes the objective character of the body through touch, it is also offers a way of alleviating any isolation experienced by an ageing person. When this occurs in the caring relationship the subjectivity of the patient is assumed to be as whole and valid as that of the carer.[37] Thus, in the act of caring the carer's focus is on the whole person who is present in bodily form.[38]

Out of this rich human conception of care come important insights. First, caring for another demands both an attitude of mind as well as effective actions towards or on behalf of the other. Second, where the notion of care has centre stage *medical care* and *cure* take subsidiary roles. Third, contemporary explorations of an ethic of care give priority to the person-centred dimensions of human caring. In this view caring is judged to be fundamentally relational such that personal responsiveness is required of the carer and, where possible, of the one to whom care is being offered. Fourth, a greater effort will have to be given to clarifying levels or degrees of care necessitated by different people in an ageing society. The moral demands of caring for others within the family context may be of a higher order than those expected of public health or community care systems. Fifth, the increasing prevalence of chronic illness in an ageing population confronts us with the reality that we will be caring for persons for whom no cure is possible. In fact a mix of health, personal and social needs will enlarge the elements of care. Whatever the need, however, the notion of care must be the central organising idea for the professional and informal modes of care offered to aged persons. Finally, the act of caring for an ageing person implies, at some point, an acknowledgment that death is inevitable and must be accepted.

The human dimensions of care just considered are greatly enriched when they are framed and transformed by the Christian understanding of *agape* or charity. Agape transforms human caring at the levels of personal motivation and personal performance. A Christian understanding of charity goes beyond the merely humanitarian dimensions of care, for an *agapeic* view of caring entails both practical solicitude for the needs of the neighbour as well as a degree of personal commitment on the part of the carer that arises from interior dispositions of mind and heart. Agape as the core of Christian care encompasses more than beneficence, philanthropy or altruism. It avoids any suggestion that care is that which occurs only between a giver and a receiver, from a greater to a lesser individual, from an expert to a lay person. Likewise in the notion of Christian care there is no limiting of care in a merely unilateral or narrowly contractual way. Rather Christian love locates care for others within the covenantal fidelity of God to human beings made concrete in his incarnate Son. An agapeic care is essentially the giving of what one has first received from God and receiving from the neighbour what God has first given to him or her.

The view that portrays health and community care as a commodity or gives undue emphasis to technical expertise and skill overlooks an essential requirement of care of the aged. Such care must be offered to aged persons by individuals who have a personal commitment and interior dispositions that shape their service of the elderly person. Without in any way diminishing the role of competence and professionalism in care of the aged agape-as-Christian-care gives priority to interpersonal relations, to the mutual interchange of equals in a community where care has a higher priority than efficiency, achievement or outcomes.

The three questions of meaning explored in the preceding pages are of central importance for an ethical evaluation of ageing in the 21st century. In the search for meaning Christians and citizens of the state are challenged to engage in a public conversation that will not only benefit the ageing members of our communities but will ultimately enhance the meaning, status and respect owed to our elders.

Questions of Justice

Age and Just Distribution of Resources

As a consequence of the serious economic down-turn that took place in the West during the early 1980s there arose in the U.S.A. a discussion as to whether age should be a criterion in distributing increasingly scarce health care resources. The bioethicist and philosopher Daniel Callahan proposed that an age criterion for access to health care might be a viable public policy initiative in a world of limited resources and ever increasing demand. His proposal of an age criterion presupposes a social value system that recognises reasonable limits. Central to Callahan's proposal is the notion that the human life-span has a natural end.[39] Medical resources should be used to help people attain their life-span. After that aged persons should only expect to receive publicly funded comfort and inexpensive treatments for acute illness.[40] In this view medical care that supports the major phases of the life cycle is understood as generating a higher moral claim than the care required to sustain life after the life cycle has been completed. The age-criterion thus functions as a mechanism for rationing health care on the basis of the natural life-span.[41]

Critics reject Callahan's proposal and claim that it is seriously flawed. His primary purpose, however, was to challenge his American society to confront the reality of limits. Callahan's ideas have been an invaluable catalyst for public discussion about the central values of American society, especially in reference to the provision of health care. Many correctly point out that it is almost impossible to reduce his thinking to a coherent public policy initiative.

The American age-criterion debate attests to widely shared concerns in Western industrialised societies about the justice issues relating to care of ageing citizens. Three consequences of this preoccupation ought be mentioned here. First, questions of justice frequently arise when human beings interact with the systems and institutions of contemporary society. More often than not this means that ageing, chronically ill and disabled persons are compelled to submit to the demands of an impersonal system. Their efforts to conform at times result in distress and disorientation arising from the failure by people working in the system to value their personal stories, capacities and preoccupations. A second concern arises from the need to scrutinise public policy from the perspective of justice. When economic rationalist considerations dominate budget thinking the matter takes on some urgency. An example of this can be seen in the changes that have taken place in Australian aged care since 1985. As part of the second wave of changes widespread restructuring has been imposed on the aged care sector throughout the Commonwealth.[42] The third wave of this reform process is expected to occur between 2008 and 2010. Should present trends continue it is fair to expect that the federal government will rely on the market place to satisfy demand for aged care services. The pivotal justice question here concerns the fairness of market forces themselves particularly when markets confront shrinking markets in a declining population.[43] A third set of justice questions may be located in discriminatory practices that ageing persons experience as a result of public neglect or the omission of those things which should be theirs by right. Ageist assumptions about an elder's ability or their right to make decisions frequently operate in the practice of care.[44] Occasions of neglect are varied such as when an elderly person falls, fractures a hip and dies while lying on the floor at home simply because there is no emergency call service provided. As community care budgets are trimmed failures of this sort will occur more frequently.

Quality-of-Life Questions

From the Christian perspective the life of a human being is a fundamental good underlying all other values. Concrete bodily existence, however, is not the highest value nor is it to be given an absolute status.[45] Christian belief in the sanctity of human life is grounded in the doctrine of God as Creator. Humankind is made in God's image with power to reason and the capacity to choose. Each individual is infinitely precious to God and made for an eternal destiny.[46]

The Christian attitude to human life can only be one of reverence. The entire Bible affirms the respect due to human life, a respect which extends to every individual from the moment of conception to extreme old age and death.[47] Human life for the Christian is a gift of God.[48] Our right to life, located as it is in our divine origin, underpins all other human rights whether they are natural or legal.[49]

A concern for *quality of life* flows from this understanding of human life.[50] A quality of life criterion commits us to weigh the values involved in each particular situation. It also enables us to discriminate among the different life-prolonging therapies available within the health care system.[51] How quality-of-life criteria are applied to issues impinging on the lives of ageing persons will be a much debated issue in the coming decades. Three problematic issues can be mentioned here.

The first is the need for individuals and society to accept the reality of death and the process of dying. Our postmodern, pluralist and secular society is a death denying one. For many of our contemporaries who have no faith in Christ death is seen only as a tragedy whose finality and inevitability is to be avoided by all means possible. Defining death as whole brain death has become increasingly problematic especially when there is increasing pressure to harvest organs for transplantation.

These developments have an effect on the way we view dying and death especially when it occurs at the end of a long life.

Physician-assisted suicide (PAS) is another contentious arena where quality-of-life is invoked. Proponents of this option emphasise a view of personal autonomy which advocates personal control of life especially of the dying process. Present criteria governing refusal of treatment, advance directives and "do not resuscitate" orders are, they claim, inadequate. Since all pain cannot be adequately controlled it is much more humane for a person who judges their life too burdensome to bring about their own death when and how they choose. This contradicts the Christian belief that killing innocent human life is morally wrong.[52] Should doctors ever be permitted to assist their patients to commit suicide our civil community will be taken onto a slippery slope where bias, greed, impatience or frustration will undermine good medical care. Vulnerable persons, especially the elderly and disabled, will find themselves under pressure to believe that their suicide is socially desirable or expected.

A third area where quality-of-life principles pose continuing challenges for medical and health care concerns questions of prolonging human life. The image of an elderly person kept alive artificially creates fear in the minds of many. Any resolution of dilemmas in this area entails confronting at least two issues. Is there a realistic hope that the patient will recover and secondly may the proposed course of action be judged to be futile? Roman Catholic moral analysis has for some time utilised the concepts of ordinary and extraordinary means to assist in clarifying what ought to be done. Where withholding or withdrawing artificial food and hydration are in question solidarity with the vulnerable and the needy must have high priority in our moral thinking. Equally significant is our awareness that nourishing another human being has great symbolic significance. As infants all of us were nourished by our mothers. In the closing days of our lives the way we nourish people speaks volumes about the type of society we seek to be.

THREE VALUES

The three sets of questions explored thus far offer an important framework for addressing many of the issues relating to ageing and ethics in the 21st century. An even more richly textured response is possible when Christians also incorporate their understandings of the human person, the solidarity that should be expressed in the human community and the range of interpersonal obligations that should bind older and younger generations together in society. It is to each of these important values that I now turn.

The Human Person: Embodied and Historical

Two aspects of the human person call for greater attention in the early decades of the new millennium. The first entails greater appreciation of the human person as *embodied*. Biblical teaching presents a unified view of the human person as both body and spirit. As the *icon* of God the body of each person is understood to be the *locus* and sacrament of healing and salvation. Such faith perspectives contribute to a valuation of human bodiliness regardless of how active or frail and limited the person may be. Historically Christianity entered a world where the body of citizens was subservient to the needs of the *polis*. Jesus' incarnation spoke of a God who reached into human existence transforming its bodily character. In the early church community the body of the martyr, the body of the monk and the body of the virgin pointed to a radical appreciation of human bodiliness arising from the gospel. Theological understandings of the sacraments as physical or bodily signs that are instruments of God's grace have contributed another rich vein of reflection on the role of the human body in salvation.[53]

A re-evaluation of human bodiliness is being pressed on the Church today from a number of different directions as diverse as *in vitro* fertilisation, sexual morality and the role of women in the Church.[54] In the past ethical analysis focused on issues relating to bodily integrity where older technologies sought to change the environment external to the human being for the *betterment* of human living. New biomedical technologies, however, seek to manipulate the internal environment *bettering* human beings.[55] In light of this dramatic change what it means to be an embodied ageing person will demand greater reflection. For not only is the body of an elderly person sacramental it must also to be touched in a healing way by the physical actions of those who care for them.

As embodied the human person is also fundamentally historical. The stories our ageing brothers and sisters love to share demands much of those who relate to them. Time and the space have to be made for the stories to be told and for people to listen to them. This is the way we express concretely our inter-connectedness with one another.

Solidarity

In an increasingly fragmented society where individualism is increasingly in evidence it is imperative that the way we live attest to the fact of our interdependence or solidarity with one another. A particular concern must be shown to the more vulnerable in our midst be they children or elderly persons. Since 1968 Roman Catholic theology has expressed this concern in terms of a *preferential option for the poor*. This perspective does not glorify poverty nor does it canonise the poor:

> it does not imply that the poor are necessarily holier than the well-heeled, that the rich and powerful are by definition evil. It involves a new way of seeing the reality in which we live, seeing it not from the standpoint of the comfortable and powerful, but from the view point of the pressured and powerless.[56]

To make an option for the poor is to commit oneself to resisting the injustice, oppression, exploitation and marginalisation of people in all areas of public life. It entails a commitment to transform society into a place where human rights and the dignity of all are respected. This option, or choice, can be made by individuals, by communities and by the whole Church.[57]

As we begin the 21st century the elderly in our midst are likely to become the new poor. This can occur in ordinary every day ways. Take for instance the locality where aged persons live. The physical dwelling and its meaning grow in importance for the individual as the years pass. Elderly people spend more time in and around the home. The comfort and conveniences of the dwelling itself, closeness to shops, public transport and other services become increasingly important as frailty and limitations increase. The home is frequently a reminder of the past, and it helps the ageing person to maintain their sense of identity and purpose through the changes of their later years. Home ownership is often the only form of wealth and evidence of status for such people. No matter where an old person lives he or she may be poor simply because of the social isolation they experience. Not only does the experience of being alone and isolated have a significant impact on an old person's health, it also says much about the texture of human interaction within our society.[58] The challenge for the future is to build interdependence between individuals, cohorts and generations such that each is enriched by a sense of belonging, community or fellowship.

Virtues

At the beginning of this paper I referred to the dependency ratio between elderly citizens and employed younger people. Alarmist messages that highlight an imbalance in dependency ratios between young and old will effectively drive a wedge between younger and older generations and pitch them into battle with each other as they compete for scarce resources. In light of this it is imperative that we consider again the relations that should exist between the generations.

Medieval theologians have offered us an analysis of the virtue of *pietas,* that virtue by which one expresses honour to one's parents, obeys and serves them.[59] The basis of this teaching in the Judaeo-Christian tradition is to be found in the decalogue command, "Honour your father and your mother."[60] Within the Jewish tradition four reasons were commonly offered as to why one must honour one's parents. First, parents are creators. The honour bestowed on parents is a continuation of the honour rendered to God. Second, there is the element of gratitude. Philo, an Alexandrian Jew and a contemporary of Jesus, located filial gratitude in the gratitude owed to benefactors. Third, proper observance of the commandment contributed to the stability of society and fourth, it ensured the preservation of the religious traditions.[61]

In the Christian context a special form of respect for old persons may be found in the spiritual friendship between them and their caregivers or between the elderly and their adult children. Housebound or bed-ridden aged persons have often outlived many of their contemporaries and frequently desire companionship more than physical care. A number of life tasks confront them. They may have a need to integrate their life experiences, cope with disengagement and loss, deal with their awareness of their limits and impending death. By listening to their stories, sharing their feelings and praying with them, family members and other caregivers can assist frail and sick old people in meeting their psychological and spiritual needs thus enriching their final years within the family network. These tasks are often quite difficult for family members and caregivers to fulfil because of the pressures arising from the demands of caring for elderly parents and their own family commitments.[62]

As mentioned earlier in this paper an understanding of responsibility is an important element in our understanding of the mutual obligations that bind families together. As people of virtue ageing persons contribute to the quality of intergenerational relations by their lives and presence. Such virtues grow through personal resolve, struggle, prayer and perseverance over a lifetime. More attention must be given to the virtues (and vices!) of old age since they form part of that intergenerational fabric that enhances (or diminishes) our social lives. William F. May has proposed that we consider the virtues of courage, humility and patience as having significance in ageing lives. Too often in the past the notion of courage has been limited to the battlefield where the prospect of death is uncertain and separation from loved ones may be only temporary. For the aged individual, on the other hand, certainty of their end and the losses entailed are anything but temporary. Aquinas described this virtue as a firmness of soul in the face of adversity. This does not result in a life free of fear or one without aversions but rather it makes possible a control of one's fears and dislikes for the sake of the good and for one's own good. Courage has a political dimension too for it calls forth in the person a readiness to make some sacrifices for the common good. The second virtue, humility, grounds the individual in an important way enabling him or her to transcend all the trials of ageing that might otherwise humiliate them. Advancing age and infirmity frequently provoke anger, frustration and bitterness. The patience of a virtuous old age does not express itself as passivity or Stoic forbearance, rather it is

> purposive waiting, receiving, willing; it demands a most intense sort of activity; it requires taking control of one's spirit precisely when all else goes out of control, when panic would send us sprawling in all directions.[63]

CONCLUSION

This paper has sketched some important aspects of ageing both of individuals and of society at the beginning of the 21st century. As this picture takes shape significant ethical issues come into focus. As a conclusion to this study, I wish to draw together the various strands in our consideration of ethics and ageing. Four important dimensions of ethical analysis as it engages the reality of human ageing in the foreseeable future merit consideration.

The first of these is the important role that context plays in any consideration of ageing and ethics. Worthwhile public analysis and discussion of ageing will progress, I have argued, only on the basis of correct demographic data and sound population projections. This information must be understood in a critical manner. Not only should there be an awareness of culturally important variants within the total population, greater attention ought also be given to the range of factors that directly have an impact on the experience of ageing. Financing retirement, access to pensions, suitable housing, transport and local amenities must complement an appropriate range of health care and welfare services. It is against this wider backdrop that ethical analysis should proceed. A diverse ethical landscape also contributes to the difficulty of any investigation. I have suggested that contemporary ethics is shaped by our postmodern age, by the pluralism of our contemporary democratic society and by the secularisation of its culture. Each of these elements contributes a level of complexity to any analysis of ageing in the 21st century. Certainly it is more likely now than in previous years that the perspective of ageing persons will have greater significance in public thinking. It will, however, be one among the many perspectives of our postmodern era. At a time when pluralist liberal society is tending to treat all as moral strangers the demands arising from the ageing of our population keep the ties of blood, family and friendship to the fore. Equally significant is the way our modern sensitivities are being blunted by a pervading secular culture. Ultimately it may only be in the struggles and the example of ageing persons that some of the transcendent issues of life will be recognised.

Public policy for an ageing society constitutes the second dimension of an ethical analysis of ageing in the 21st century. In an era when there is a heightened awareness that our ecosystem is being imperilled by industrial development and its attendant pollution it is to be expected that scarce resources and their allocation should be on the public agenda. The courageous effort by Daniel Callahan to provoke debate about the reality of limits in social life must be applauded. His intent was to reverse some of the side-effects of increasing dependence on technology and technological solutions in American society. His notion of an age criterion may prove to be inadequate as a suitable public policy option for the delivery of health care to persons in their latter years. Nevertheless, the issue will not go away. Limited and even scarce resources are forcing us to face the fact that choices must be made and that not everything that can be done ought to be done particularly in the area of health care delivery and welfare services. It would be a great benefit to public policy development if a broad ranging discussion of resources and their use could be undertaken across the nation. This would enable some consensus on the place and roles of all age cohorts in society. A consequence of this might be a greater appreciation of ageing and aged persons. Unfortunately, because our ethical approach is permeated by postmodern concerns and ethical pluralism there is little likelihood that a real consensus could be achieved. Any ethical analysis of resource allocation during the coming decades must necessarily surface the valuation of individuals, groups and age cohorts lurking below the surface. The end result may be a better appreciation of ageing and aged persons in society.

To progress a public conversation on ageing greater emphasis will have to be given to skills of reflection and styles of explanation. This constitutes the third dimension of an ethical analysis as it addresses the phenomenon of human ageing. Questions of meaning, especially the three explored earlier in this paper, demand an ability to reflect at some depth. Our individual and community capacity to reflect is frequently muted by an over concentration on data or concrete phenomena. In searching for an answer to the meaning of ageing, well-being and care I have given priority to the significance of human experience, cultural and historical understandings and the theological approaches of Christianity. Perhaps what is needed more than ever in contemporary public discourse is a disciplined and consistent reflection by all the participants in the conversation. This entails a greater level of skill and commitment to reflection. Equally important is a level of openness to the wide range of humanistic and theological explanations that history and contemporary experience offer about human ageing. These two elements, namely skills of reflection and styles of explanation, will ensure a more comprehensive approach to ethics and the issues of ageing in the decades ahead.

For an ageing society the core ethical issues at the beginning of the 21st century hinge on the meaning of human life and the ways we evaluate it. This is the fourth dimension of an ethical analysis of ageing. The quality-of-life issues briefly considered in this paper–dying and death, physician-assisted suicide and the challenges of prolonging human life–attest to the core nature and value of human life. The variety of responses in our secular, postmodern and pluralist society to the demands of individual human beings be they newborn infants, disabled children or active or chronically ill elderly persons poses this value question with greater urgency than before. That we are able to choose and technically implement decisions in ever more sophisticated ways calls into question our ethical analysis and the value we place on human existence in the new millennium. In the latter part of this paper I suggested three perspectives on human life that have a direct bearing on ageing and the lives of aged persons. In valuing the human person priority must necessarily be given to the physical, embodied reality of the individual and the unique narrative that is his or her life. By emphasising human solidarity an ethically justifiable preference is given to those who are marginalised in society. Unless ageing is re-evaluated in contemporary Australian society in the reflective way suggested above there is a real possibility that aged persons will be marginalised in society and become the "new poor." Furthermore, in the virtues (and vices) of aged persons and the relations between them and their children there arises a need to examine the quality of presence human beings have one to another. Not only is this significant in family relationships it is also vital for care and support for everyone in the wider community.

The four dimensions of context, public policy, reflection and the value of human life just outlined constitute pivotal issues for ethical analysis of ageing in the 21st century.

NOTES

1. H. Mackay, *Turning Point. Australians Choosing Their Future.* (Sydney: Macmillan, 1999), 76.

2. House of Representatives Standing Committee for Long Term Strategies, *Expectations of Life. Increasing the Options for the 21st Century,* (Canberra: Australian Government Publishing Service, 1992), 22-24.

3. D.T. Rowland, *Ageing in Australia. Population Trends and Social Issues,* (Melbourne: Longman Cheshire, 1992), 25.

4. J. McCallum & K. Geiselhart, *Australia's New Aged. Issues for Young and Old,* (Sydney: Allen & Unwin, 1996), 7.

5. Mackay, xix.

6. Mackay, xx. See also P. Lakeland, *Postmodernity. Christian Identity in a Fragmented Age,* (Minneapolis: Fortress Press, 1997).

7. McCallum & Geiselhart, 16.

8. R. Gascoigne, *Freedom and Purpose. An Introduction to Christian Ethics,* (Sydney: E.J. Dwyer, 1993), 10.

9. Gascoigne, 14.

10. H.T. Engelhardt, *Bioethics and Secular Humanism. The Search for a Common Morality,* (London: SCM Press, 1991), 96-101, 121-124.

11. Cf. J. Bowker (ed.), *The Oxford Dictionary of World Religions,* (New York: Oxford University Press, 1997), "secularization," 871-872.

12 John 1:14.

13. M.P. Gallagher, "From Social to Cultural Secularization," *Louvain Studies,* 24 (1999): 113.

14. Gallagher, 104.

15. Gallagher, 105.

16. D.C. Thomasma, "Professional and Ethical Obligations Toward the Aged," *The Linacre Quarterly* 48:1 (1981): 74-75.

17. D.S. Browning, "Preface to a Practical Theology of Ageing" in *Toward a Theology of Ageing,* edited by S. Hiltner, (New York: Human Sciences Press, 1975), 154-155.

18. S.A. Gadow, "Frailty and Strength: The Dialectic of Ageing" In *What Does It Mean to Grow Old? Reflections from the Humanities,* edited by T.R. Cole and S. Gadow, (Durham, N.C.: Duke University Press, 1986), 238.

19. Cf. T.R. Cole, *The Journey of Life. A Cultural History of Ageing in America,* (Cambridge: Cambridge University Press, 1992), xviii.

20. Cf. D. Leder, *The Absent Body,* (Chicago: University of Chicago Press, 1990).

21. D. Leder, "Health and Disease. V. The Experience of Health and Illness," in *Encyclopedia of Bioethics,* edited by W.T. Reich, (New York: Simon & Schuster Macmillan, 1995), II, 1108-1109.

22. E. Scarry, *The Body in Pain: The Making and Unmaking of the World,* (New York: Oxford University Press, 1985), 35.

23. L.H. Landon, "Suffering Over Time: Six Varieties of Pain", *Soundings* 72:1 (1989): 75.

24. Kimble, "Religion: Friend or Foe of the Aging?" *Second Opinion,* 15 (1990): 74.

25. Job 42:1-6.

26. P.S. Keane, *Health Care Reform. A Catholic View,* (New York: Paulist Press, 1993), 66.

27. Cf. X. Leon-Dufour (ed.), *Dictionary of Biblical Theology,* (London: Geoffrey Chapman, 1984), 586-590.

28. Mt. 9:36; 14:14; 15:32; cf. Jn. 11.

29. 2 Cor.1:5.

30. Rom 8:17; 2 Cor.4:10.

31. Phil.1:29; cfl. Ac.9:16; 2 Cor.11:23-27.

32. 2 Cor.4:17; cf. Ac.14:21; 2 Cor.7:4; cf. Ac.5:41; 1 Pt.4:13-14.

33. Col.1:24.

34. Anglo-American philosophical texts give scant attention to pain and suffering; no articles are to be found in the *Encyclopedia of Philosophy* and *The Oxford Companion to Philosophy.*

35. Cf. E. J. Cassel, "The Nature of Suffering and the Goals of Medicine," *The New England Journal of Medicine* (1982): 640-643.

36. Cf. Keane, *Health Care Reform,* 81.

37. Cf. S. Gadow, "Nurse and Patient: The Caring Relationship" in *Caring, Curing, Coping. Nurse, Physician, Patient Relationships,* edited by A.H. Bishop and J.R. Scudder, (Alabama: University of Alabama Press, 1985), 31-43.

38. Cf. R.A. McCormick, "Some Neglected Aspects of the Moral Responsibility for Health" in *How Brave a New World? Dilemmas in Bioethics,* (London: S.C.M. Press, 1981), 43.

39. Cf. K.M. Dixon, "Oppressive Limits: Callahan's Foundation Myth," *The Journal of Medicine and Philosophy* 19 (1994): 617-619.

40. D. Callahan, *Setting Limits. Medical Goals in an Aging Society,* (New York: Simon & Schuster, 1987), 116.

41. Cf. G. R. Winslow, "Exceptions and the Elderly" in *Facing Limits. Ethics and Health Care for the Elderly,* edited by G.R. Winslow and J.W. Walters, (Boulder, CO: Westview Press, 1993), 236-37.

42. The "Aged Care Structural Reform" was introduced by the coalition government in 1997.

43. R. Gray, "The Third Wave of Aged Care Reforms," *Health Matters* 3 (1999): 10-12.

44. McCallum and Geiselhart, 25.

45. W.T. Reich, "Life, Prolongation of" in *A New Dictionary of Christian Ethics,* edited by J. F. Childress and J. Macquarrie, (London: SCM Press, 1986), 351.

46. T. Wood, "Life, Sacredness of" in *A New Dictionary of Christian Ethics,* edited by J. F. Childress and J. Macquarrie, (London: SCM Press, 1986), 353.

47. Ex.20:13; Dt.5:17: "You shall not kill." The prophets refer to the crime of shedding innocent blood (Is.59:7; Jer.22:3; Ez.22:4). In Mt.5:21-26 Jesus extends respect for human life to the inner dispositions of hatred and anger. Paul sees the prohibition against murder as being present in the consciences of all human beings, be they believers or not (Rom.1:29-32).

48. Cf. S.T. II-II, 64, a.4 and a.6.

49. Cf. T.D. Whitmore, "Human Rights" in *The HarperCollins Encyclopedia of Catholicism,* edited by R.P. McBrien, (New York: HarperCollins, 1995), 643-44.

50. For a review of the literature see L.S. Cahill, "Notes on Moral Theology: 1986. Sanctity of Life, Quality of Life, and Social Justice," *Theological Studies* 48 (1987): 105-14.

51. Keane, *Health Care Reform,* 73-74.

52. *Catechism of the Catholic Church,* (Sydney: St. Pauls, 1994), nn.2276-2279.

53. K. Rahner, "The Body in the Order of Salvation" in *Theological Investigations,* (London: Darton, Longman and Todd, 1981), vol. 17, 71-78.

54. Cf. R. Brungs, "Biology and the Future: A Doctrinal Agenda," *Theological Studies* 50 (1989): 700.

55. Brungs, "Biology . . . ," 702-703.

56. W. Burghardt, "Characteristics of Social Justice Spirituality", *Origins* 24:9 (1994): 160-161.

57. D. Dorr, "Poor, Preferential Option for" in *The New Dictionary of Catholic Social Thought,* edited by J.A. Dwyer and E.L. Montgomery, (Collegeville, Minn.: The Liturgical Press, 1994), 755; for a theological analysis of the option for the poor see J. O'Brien, *Theology and the Option for the Poor,* (Collegeville, Minn.: The Liturgical Press, 1992).

58. McCallum and Geiselhart, 100.

59. Cf. T.O. Martin, "Piety, Familial" in *New Catholic Encyclopedia,* (New York: McGraw-Hill, 1967), vol. 11, 356-358; for a philosophical analysis of the notion *pietas* see D. Walhout, "Piety, Value, and Culture" in *The Good and the Realm of Values,* (Notre Dame, Ind.: University of Notre Dame Press, 1978), 21-38.

60. Ex.20:12. Cf. R.F. Collins, "The Fourth Commandment–For Children or for Adults?" in *Christian Morality: Biblical Foundations,* (Notre Dame, Ind.: University of Notre Dame Press, 1986), 89.

61. G. Blidstein, *Honor Thy Father and Mother. Filial Responsibility in Jewish Law and Ethics,* (New York: KTAV Publishing, 1975), 1-36.

62. D. Christiansen, "Creative Social Responses to Ageing. Public Policy Options for Family Caregiving" in *Concilium,* edited by L.S. Cahill and D. Mieth, (London: SCM Press, 1991), 117, 119-121.

63. W.F. May, "The Virtues and Vices of the Elderly," in *What Does It mean to Grow Old?* edited by T.R. Cole and S.A. Gadow, (Durham: Duke University Press, 1986), 52.

Beyond the Biomedical Paradigm: Generating a Spiritual Vision of Ageing

Melvin A. Kimble, PhD

SUMMARY. The time has come to enlarge our understanding of what an ageing older person truly is. What is called for is an approach to ageing and its multiple processes that moves beyond an empirical research model, which is limited to a positivistic focus on the bio-medical and social conditions of ageing. The spiritual dimension of the individual as well as the physical and social need to be acknowledged and valued in any definition of human existence. A segmental approach to the ageing process can only result on a reductionistic, one-dimensional caricature of the older person. There is an imperative need for the inclusion of the spiritual dimension in the study of ageing and its meaning. By issuing a call for a new wholistic paradigm that moves beyond the bio-medical model, and understanding the personhood is affirmed which includes a person's capacity to find meaning in life, indeed, even in ageing, suffering and dying. *[Article copies available for a fee from The Haworth Document Delivery Service: 1-800-342-9678. E-mail address: <getinfo@haworthpressinc.com> Website: <http://www.HaworthPress.com> © 2001 by The Haworth Press, Inc. All rights reserved.]*

KEYWORDS. Biomedical paradigm, dimensional ontology, dying and death, gero-transcendence, meaning, spiritual/spirituality, suffering, symbols

Melvin A. Kimble is Professor Emeritus of Pastoral Theology, Luther Seminary, Director of the Center for Aging, Religion and Spirituality, St. Paul, MN.

[Haworth co-indexing entry note]: "Beyond the Biomedical Paradigm Generating a Spiritual Vision of Ageing." Kimble, Melvin A. Co-published simultaneously in *Journal of Religious Gerontology* (The Haworth Pastoral Press, an imprint of The Haworth Press, Inc.) Vol. 12, No. 3/4, 2001, pp. 31-41; and: *Aging, Spirituality and Pastoral Care: A Multi-National Perspective* (ed: Elizabeth MacKinlay, James W. Ellor, and Stephen Pickard) The Haworth Pastoral Press, an imprint of The Haworth Press, Inc., 2001, pp. 31-41. Single or multiple copies of this article are available for a fee from The Haworth Document Delivery Service [1-800-342-9678, 9:00 a.m. - 5:00 p.m. (EST). E-mail address: getinfo@haworthpressinc.com].

One of the great surprises of the twentieth century was the gift of longer life. Never before in the history of humankind has the average life expectancy increased so dramatically. This extended life expectancy with its noisy ticking of the biological clock has resulted in an emerging danger of identifying the whole process of ageing through a biomedical lens.

STAGES OF GERONTOLOGY

There are historical reasons why gerontology and the study of ageing have evolved emphasizing the bio-medical dimensions. Physicians and biologists were the first to study ageing with the result that a biomedical paradigm became the lens, which has shaped and generally defined how ageing and growing old are viewed. Consequently this is the lens through which persons perceived the chronological passing of time and the concomitant changes in their bodies. Although it is true that in the second stage in the study of gerontology, psychologists and sociologists along with economists and demographers began seriously to examine ageing and its processes, the bio-medical paradigm continued to dominate our understanding of ageing. The result of this bio-medical model is the "medicalization" of ageing which has been perpetuated in our society.

The contemporary concept of "successful ageing" has been introduced into current discourse concerning older adulthood.[1] It implies that if one can pass for ten years younger than he or she actually is, maintain a low cholesterol reading and blood pressure level, or move about a tennis court with some agility; or pass the treadmill stress test–then one has satisfied the criteria for "successful ageing" and, subsequently, a longer life expectancy. That is what living is all about, isn't it? Longevity is the point, right? Wrong! Has any culture so obsessed by long life and extended years ever been in such denial as well as fear about ageing and becoming older? This has resulted in a gerontophobic attitude towards ageing and the chronological passing of time. All of this generates a particular glorification of youthfulness and an irrational denial of the natural life processes of ageing and dying.

One might speculate that at the basis of the fear of ageing is the fear of the ultimate life event, which is death. In spite of the euphemistic promise of the recent discovery of an "immortality enzyme" that encourages cells to keep dividing indefinitely, and anti-ageing medicine proponents that prophesy that we may even see "practical immortality" within our lifetime, life moves inexorably towards death. Over fifteen hundred years ago, Augustine understood this well and stated:

For no sooner do we begin to live in this dying body, than we begin to move ceaselessly towards death. For in the whole course of this life (if life we must call it) its mutability tends toward death . . . For whatever time we live is deducted from our whole term of life, and that which remains is daily becoming less and less; so that our whole life is nothing but a race towards death, in which no one is allowed to stand still for a little space, or to go somewhat more slowly, but all are driven forwards with an impartial movement, and with equal rapidity.[2]

T. S. Eliot suggested there are two basic questions in life: namely, *What are we going to do about it? and What does it mean?* The biomedical paradigm has in many respects served gerontology well by answering the first question. We have all been beneficiaries of not only extended life expectancy, but also of improved health with which we live out these additional years. This model, however, is powerless to answer the second question, *What does it mean?* The bio-medical paradigm is not hermeneutically nor philosophically equipped to explore and create new dimensions for understanding the meaning of growing and being old. It has been observed that

Since World War II, a vast empirical literature of gerontology has grown up. The dominant methodology in that literature has been inspired by a positivistic view of the natural and social sciences, a view that makes it difficult even to think of meaning as a legitimate object of inquiry.[3]

Most of the research, which has been conducted in the study of ageing, is based on a positivistic paradigm and has utilized the quantitative approach, which has excluded the spiritual dimension.

CALL FOR A NEW PARADIGM

What is lacking is a concern for hermeneutics, not simply medical statistics; for understanding, not simply diagnosis and prognosis. A new paradigm is required which confronts and interprets the negativities and the inevitable diminishments and losses of older adulthood with its narrowing boundaries. All of this calls for a *third stage* of gerontology which enlarges and enriches the understanding of the ageing process and introduces a wholistic and inclusive model which views the aged person beyond the bio-medical and psychosocial models. Throughout life, at every stage, the developing self is confronted with the necessity of making interpretations and assigning meanings to what has been and is being experienced.

It has been observed that the enormous gains in longevity through medical and technological progress have been accompanied " . . . by a widespread spiritual malaise . . . over the meaning and purpose of human life–particularly in old age."[4] This experience of a sense of emptiness and meaninglessness has been discovered in the elderly populations of industrialized nations.[5] Such global statistics seem to confirm Viktor Frankl's observation that "The truth is that as the struggle for survival has subsided, the question has emerged: *survival for what?* Ever more people today have the means to live but no meaning to live for."[6] For many it appears that the crisis of old age is a crisis of meaning. The ultimate answer would be for old age itself to offer the elderly something worthwhile for which to live. Meaning-making at its core is a spiritual exercise.

Once the validity of the spiritual dimension has been acknowledged a whole new world of interpretation of ageing and growing old opens up. Old questions concerning the meaning of this last stage of the life cycle and its accompanying questions of suffering and dying come to take on a multivalent quality that is multidimensional in its examination of ageing and growing old.

FRANKL'S DIMENSIONAL ONTOLOGY

It is specifically at this point that Viktor Frankl's logotherapy makes an important, indeed essential contribution to helping persons probe the meaning of ageing. Frankl contends that any examination of ageing and the ageing process should reflect an understanding that it is the whole person who is ageing and aged. This whole is a dynamic blend of spiritual, physical, mental, emotional and social dimensions of human personhood. The spiritual dimension of the individual as well, as well as the physical and social dimensions need to be acknowledged and valued in any definition of authentic human existence. A segmental approach to the ageing process will only result in a reductionistic, one-dimensional caricature of the older person.

In order to avoid the Cartesian body-mind dualism, Frankl developed what he referred to as "dimensional ontology." His system of psychotherapy, called logotherapy, adds to the somatic and the psychic dimensions of the person an emphasis on the third dimension, namely, the spiritual dimension; or as Frankl preferred to label it, the *noetic* dimension. This dimension–in contradistinction to the biological or psychological dimension–is the dimension in which the uniquely human phenomena are located. As Frankl suggests, it could be defined as the spiritual dimension.

The geometrical concept of dimensional ontology set forth by Frankl recognizes the rich and varied multi-dimensionality of individuals while still preserving their anthropological unity. Frankl demonstrated this by the following example:

> . . . A glass on the table, if projected out of three-dimensional space into a two-dimensional plane, would appear as a circle. The same glass projected into its side view and seen in profile would appear as a rectangle. But nobody would claim that the glass is composed of a circle and a rectangle. Neither can claim that man is composed of parts, such as a body and a soul. It is a violation of man to project him out of the realm of the genuinely human in the plane of either soma or psyche.[7]

The meaning of human existence extends beyond the plane of merely psychodynamic or psychogenetic, e.g., MMP profile or DNA strand. As Frankl urged, we must follow a person " . . . into the dimension of the specifically human phenomena that is the spiritual dimension of being."[8] Dimensional ontology widens that lens through which we perceive older persons and their ageing process.

Healthcare providers and policy makers as well as gerontological researchers are expanding their conception of well-being in later life. What has been missing in healthcare is being described as spirituality. It has been acknowledged that there is something to be learned from the way in which spirituality and religion help people to adjust to and cope with some of the distressing and burdensome aspects of older adulthood. The spiritual (*geistig*) is the energy within a person that strives for meaning and purpose. It is the unifying and integrating dimension of being that includes the experience of transcendence and the mystery of the holy. That mystery is at once overwhelming and fascinating, but renders existence significant and meaningful. The term spirituality describes this timeless and universal search for meaning and the desire for wholeness and an awareness of the presence of the numinous.

The spiritual dimension is increasingly being recognized as the most important dimension in healthcare today. It is gaining recognition as a critical component to "successful ageing." It appears that the time has come to enlarge our understanding of what an older person truly is–the essence of one's very being. The key to answering the urgent question, *Is growing old worth one's whole life to attain?* can be discovered within the parameters of the exploration of this third paradigm.

SYMBOLS OF TRANSCENDENCE

There is an absence of symbols of transcendence in our society that would enable persons to discover answers to questions related to the meaning of ageing and growing old. Symbols provide guideposts for persons as they move into the future, even into dying and death. A true symbol moves beyond itself, not only denoting something, but also suggesting that which is hidden. The hiddeness is not just buried in the past, but also contains a promise of the future. It captures the undiscovered "more" to which a symbol always points. It never simply escapes into the past, but always opens into the future. The ability to symbolize allows persons to transcend time boundaries, to reminisce about the past and to anticipate the future. By symbolization, persons are able to interpret and articulate the meaning of their existence. As they pass through time, they formulate all of the events of their lives and construct their "lived world" of meanings.

Devoid of transcendent symbols that facilitate acceptance and give meaning to the natural process of ageing and dying, persons frantically search for deliverance in the latest medical messiah. The present crisis of meaning calls for relevant symbols and rituals that sustain and extend meaning as individuals live out their lives.

An examination of ageing from the perspective of Judeo-Christian tradition explores the human dimensions and contours of the ageing experience. It probes the interior as well as the exterior dynamics of the ageing process. The goal is to examine the unique personal experiences of ageing with its increasingly narrowing boundaries and the cascade of changes and losses that mark one's passage through life. It includes those occasions in which God's love most poignantly interfaces with a person's life and when a sense of life's ultimate meaning is introduced. The faith tradition has an extraordinary opportunity to claim a primary role as an affirmer of the value and worth of all persons at every stage of life and to become a generator of personal and social meanings. In a society that measures the value of life in ways that often de-value and de-humanize, the religious sector with its recreative power confronts persons at whatever stage with a destiny and a purpose.

An impoverished symbol system results in expressions of guilt without absolution, of isolation and alienation which have forgotten the covenant promise and relationship, as well as their expression in the household of faith and of suffering that is void of meaning and only devalues and debases the sufferer. The sacred writings of different religions with their symbols and rites speak of the meaning of life and the meaning of death, of the mysteries of evil and suffering, as well as the mysteries of love and healing. Judaism, as Katz clarifies, "promises no simple salvation, but at the same time it is rooted in a deep belief that God is the God of life."[9] The salvific symbols and rites of the Christian faith tradition and practice provide powerful sources of meanings in centering the existential order of life. The cross, for example, is a powerful symbol of meaning fashioned out of suffering. The Jewish and Christian traditions probe the interior as well as the exterior dynamics of the aging process. They speak to the deepest substrata of our being. They involve all of our nature–the senses, feelings, memory and mind. In this encounter with the symbolic, our fragmented selves may be healed and reconstructed. The introduction of such symbols of meaning in the midst of suffering and ageing, does not deny reality, but rather transcends it. This includes examining those occasions in which God's love most poignantly interfaces with a person's life and a sense of ultimate meaning is introduced.

The wisdom of the historic Jewish and Christian traditions offer guidance as we face the avalanche of pre-mortem questions that have been introduced by present healthcare and longer life expectancy. Human life is understood to be God's gift to be lived with thanksgiving. This life, however, is not absolute. It is not for itself; it is given for the purpose of glorifying God and serving one's neighbor.

The different religious traditions are sources to assist older adults who struggle with issues of integrity and meaning by providing them access to the rich heritage of symbols and rites through which persons understand their relationship to God, the source of ultimate meaning. Theologian David Tracy suggests that symbols can orient us positively for the process of ageing:

> What is fundamentally at stake . . . is but a reverence for ourselves as a part of nature and a respect for the diversity of that temporal, aging self in such a manner that the integrity or dignity of every human being is affirmed without qualification. The Judeo-Chris-

tian symbol system, I believe, can disclose precisely that reverence and illuminate that dignity. Theological reflection, therefore, may provide something like a horizon of meaningfulness, an orientation to the value of aging that may serve to clarify and strengthen the specific analysis found by the sciences.[10]

GERO-TRANSCENDENCE

This new paradigm that includes the spiritual dimension of life results in a radically new understanding of questions concerning the meaning of ageing. It introduces what Lars Tornstan, a representative from the human sciences, describes as a "time of gero-transcendence in which individuals gradually experience a new understanding of fundamental existential questions–often a cosmic communion with the spirit of the universe and a redefinition of the self and relationships with others."[11] Tornstan continues: " . . . Simply put, gero-transcendence is a shift in meta-perspective, from a materialistic and pragmatic view of the world to a more cosmic and transcendent one."[12]

Frankl believes that self-transcendence is the essence of human existence. He explains:

> I thereby understand the primordial anthropological fact that being human is being always directed and pointing to something or someone other than oneself: to a meaning to fulfill or another human being to encounter, a cause to serve or a person to love. Only to the extent that someone is living out this self-transcendence of human existence, is he truly human or does he become his true self. He becomes so, not by concerning with self with his self's actualization, but by forgetting himself and giving himself, overlooking himself and focusing outward.[13]

Until the very end of life, the older person has both actuality and potentiality–the ability to transcend the present situation and to see one's capacity to alter the status quo, even if limited to one's own attitude toward unavoidable suffering. Potentialities for meaning are ever present in life. Neither suffering nor dying can detract from them. There is a need to challenge the reductionistic approach and to recognize that the meaning of suffering may well be hidden in another dimension beyond the bodily symptomatology.

SPIRITUAL THICKNESS

Alternative images and metaphors are required in which ageing is not simply regarded as loss and diminution, but becomes a time of spiritual enlargement and fulfillment. Ann Belford Ulanov sets forth her view of the spiritual task of aging:

> Aging brings home to us what we have done or failed to do with our lives, our creativity or our waste, our openness to zealous hiding from what really matters. Precisely at that point, age cracks us open, sometimes for the first time, makes us aware of the center, makes us look for it and for relation to it. Aging does not mark an end but rather beginning of making sense of the end-questions, so that life can have an end in every sense of the word.[14]

In order to confront the questions and challenges of older adulthood, a person must be girded by a "thickness" of spiritual resources. In other words, the transition to older adulthood must first be made in the spiritual dimension. Perhaps the failure to do this is what makes it so difficult to cross the border from middle age into older adulthood. Maybe persons are fearful that God will not accompany them into this strange unexplored terrain. Older adulthood needs a continuing vision of God and God's kingdom and an individual's place in it. What does it mean, for example, to grow old under the promises of the love of God? What does God have in mind for persons in the last stage of the life-cycle? What are the resources within one's religious tradition that make the later years of life's journey a new adventure of grace?

Such questions test one's spiritual thickness to the limit. Old age is not the ideal stage for the creation *de nova* of spiritual maturity. Persons must, however, begin from whatever level of spiritual development they bring to the last stage of life. Spiritual maturation is the developmental task that confronts the final stage of life.

Our spirituality is an opening out from space and time–a window that discloses a destiny inextricably tied to mystery. There is no way for a human being to understand fully himself or herself other than in terms of transcendence. Human persons are persons only to the extent that they understand themselves, *sub specie aeternitatus,* under the aspect of eternity. Ageing is a singular way to see ourselves in the image of God.

For the Christian, the Gospel is the good news about ageing and dying and growing old. In a society that measures the value of life in ways that often devalue and dehumanize, the Gospel, with its recreative power, confronts a person with a destiny and a purpose. The center of gravity for shared human life in time is not an internalized past, but the promise and power of an astonishing gracious new future already coming toward humanity and all creation.

It is such an understanding of the transcendent mystery of God's love that envelopes life, and that enables one to let loose of life in the death event with the same peaceful and confident faith that Roman Catholic theologian Karl Rahner confessed shortly before his death at the age of 80:

> The real high point of my life is still to come. I mean the abyss of the mystery of God into which one lets oneself fall in complete confidence of being caught up by God's love and mercy forever.[15]

CONCLUSION

We live in a society where ageing is often viewed as an embarrassment, suffering and dying a meaningless experience and death a medical failure. Older adults find themselves stranded in the unchartered territory of longer life expectancy with a pervasive bio-medical model of ageing, void of sacramental meaning. Suffering from biological angst as a result of living in a body that daily reflects its planned obsolescence, older persons are often reduced to preoccupation about their changing bodies. There is no denying that ageing is built into one's physiology.

As James Hillman points out, "to *explain* ageing, we usually turn to biology, genetics and geriatric physiology, but to understand ageing we need something *more*,"[16] what is urgently required is a new paradigm that offers "something more"–images and understandings, symbols and rituals that provide a transcendent meaning of life conveyed by an Ultimate Being. This is a paradigm that recognizes the spiritual dimension as the inclusive and encompassing dimension for understanding and integrating the ageing experience. It circumscribes that which is not comprehensible in biology, psychology and other scientific disciplines.

In issuing such a call for a new wholistic paradigm, care must be taken to avoid the Scylla of biologism or the equally dangerous Charybdis of spiritualizing the ageing process. By emphasizing that a human being is not simply a psychosomatic organism, this new paradigm moves beyond the bio-medical model and introduces a wholistic understanding of personhood which affirms one's capacity to find meaning in life, indeed, even in ageing, suffering and dying. It is this unique spiritual capacity, which conveys a fresh awareness of self-worth and human dignity and enables persons to understand and perceive themselves as fashioned in the image of God and to believe that there is a transcendent destiny built into this transitory life.

NOTES

1. John W. Rowe and Robert L. Kahn, *Successful Aging,* (New York: Pantheon Books, 1999), 38.

2. W. J. Oates, *Basic Writing of St. Augustine,* (New York: Random House, 1948), 217.

3. Harry R. Moody and Thomas R. Cole, "Aging and Meaning: A Bibliographical Essay," Eds. Thomas R. Cole and Sally A. Gadow, *What Does it Mean to Grow Old,* (Durham: Duke University Press, 1986), 248.

4. Thomas R. Cole, "Aging, Meaning, and Well-Being: Musings of a Cultural Historian," *International Journal of Aging and Human Development,* 19, (1984), 329.

5. Hiroshi Takashima, *Psychomatic Medicine and Logotherapy,* (Oceanside, New York: Dabor Science Publication, 1977), 60.

6. Viktor Frankl, *The Unheard Cry for Meaning.* (New York: Simon & Schuster, 1979), 21.

7. Viktor Frankl, *Psychotherapy and Existentialism,* Selected Papers on Logotherapy, (New York: The World Publishing Company, 1969, Paperback Edition, New York: New American Library, 1976), 138.

8. Ibid., 73.

9. R. L. Katz, *Pastoral Care and the Jewish Tradition,* (Philadelphia: Fortress Press, 1985), 178.

10. David Tracy, "Eschatological Perspectives on Aging." In Seward Hiltner's *Toward a Theology of Aging.* (New York: Human Sciences Press, 1975), 133.

11. Lars Tornstan, "Gerortranscendence in a Broad Cross-Sectional Perspective, *Journal of Aging and Identity,* Vol. 2, No. l, 1977.

12. Ibid.

13. Frankl, *The Unheard Cry for Meaning,* 35.

14. Ann Belford Ulanov, "Aging: On the Way to One's End." In Clements, W., ed., *Ministry with the Aging,* (New York: Harper and Row, 1981), 122.

15. Karl Rahner, *Faith in a Wintry Season: Conversations and Interviews With Karl Rahner in the Last Years of his Life.* Edited by Paul Imhof and Hubert Bullowans. Trans. & ed. Harvey D. Egan. (New York: Crossroad, 1990), 38.

16. James Hillman, *The Force of Character and the Lasting Life,* (New York: Random House, 1999), xiv.

Outward Decay and Inward Renewal: A Biblical Perspective on Aging and the Image of God

John Painter, PhD

SUMMARY. We read in the Christian scriptures that length of life is a blessing from the Lord. However, with age comes physical decline and other social problems which today make this a mixed blessing. Yet there is a promise of the renewal of the inner person, day by day even though the cracked and decaying earthen vessel remains. The challenge is to find those aspects of life which are renewed by the gospel. The restoration of the *image* of God puts the focus on the restored relationship to God for which humans were created and the consequent renewal of relationship with each other. As we grow older, we need to struggle to maintain this perspective. *[Article copies available for a fee from The Haworth Document Delivery Service: 1-800-342-9678. E-mail address: <getinfo@haworthpressinc.com> Website: <http://www.HaworthPress.com> © 2001 by The Haworth Press, Inc. All rights reserved.]*

KEYWORDS. Spirit, decay, soul, renewal, relationship, *imago dei,* earthen vessels, transformation

John Painter is Professor of Theology, School of Theology, Charles Sturt University, Australia.

[Haworth co-indexing entry note]: "Outward Decay and Inward Renewal: A Biblical Perspective on Aging and the Image of God." Painter, John. Co-published simultaneously in *Journal of Religious Gerontology* (The Haworth Pastoral Press, an imprint of The Haworth Press, Inc.) Vol. 12, No. 3/4, 2001, pp. 43-55; and: *Aging, Spirituality and Pastoral Care: A Multi-National Perspective* (ed: Elizabeth MacKinlay, James W. Ellor, and Stephen Pickard) The Haworth Pastoral Press, an imprint of The Haworth Press, Inc., 2001, pp. 45-55. Single or multiple copies of this article are available for a fee from The Haworth Document Delivery Service [1-800-342-9678, 9:00 a.m. - 5:00 p.m. (EST). E-mail address: getinfo@haworthpressinc.com].

My task is to give a biblical perspective on aging and spirituality. Two things learned during the second half of the twentieth century need brief comment at this point. First, the Bible embodies a diversity of views. Hence all I can offer is *a* Biblical perspective. In this case, for a variety of reasons, I have chosen a Pauline perspective. The simplest of the reasons is that, when I was asked to give the paper the text that underlies my title instantly popped into my mind. Reflection added weightier reasons.[1] Second, we have become more clearly aware that *our situation* or *context* affects our *point of view,* that is, the way we look at anything, including the Bible.

Thus there is a need to take account of our *context* and the way it influences our understanding of a Biblical view. We need to do this anyway, because the purpose of the Biblical perspective in this conference is to throw light on the *problems* and *possibilities* of aging, spirituality and pastoral care today. If we fail to take the initiative in grasping the opportunities in our own unique and evolving context we will be left only with the problems, wallowing in unavoidable crises.

There is a tendency today to regard older people as "past it," worth*less*. Even in the past there is evidence of economic rationalism (see Leviticus 27), a tendency to regard older people as worth*less*. This is partly a consequence of the failure to value wisdom and experience. It is also a confusion of what we are, with what we do, which is not difficult to explain because the two, though not identical, are closely related. Yet, in the long run, it is important to remember the distinction because human value and destiny in God's purpose find expression in understanding the "image of God."

At the same time there are many good reasons for older people in good health to extend their working lives. By extending the working life, social links that might otherwise be lost are maintained. The importance of maintaining a life that is characterized by connection with other people and with a concern for the needs of others is something I want to stress in relation to spirituality and its benefit for those growing older.

Experience is something that older people have in plenty, as is tested judgement though this can be made ineffective by growing caution and fearfulness. Certainly memory is a complex faculty. Some aspects are more seriously affected at earlier stages of aging than others are and aging is not uniform in all people, as the Victoria Longitudinal Studies (VLS) have shown.[2] Yet the very old can often remember the past quite remarkably when patience and care is taken to explore their memories. Thus there is a need for us to recognize which faculties can be developed and enhanced with age without becoming frustrated by the loss of what seems to be inevitably diminished in aging. So we come to my main theme.

Taking my cue from Paul I have entitled the paper: *Outward Decay and Inward Renewal: A Biblical Perspective on Aging and the Image of God.* This leads to the question, "What does spirituality contribute in the context of aging?" My approach is to use Paul as a way into this theme. Paul draws on a Jewish anthropology but has modified it in significant ways in the light of his faith in the Christ and his own maturing experience. Briefly, Paul accepts the earthiness of human life, created from the dust of the earth. But with the breath of God, the human is a living person. The word translated as "soul" (ψυχή) means, in this context, a living person. Notice Genesis 2:7 says, "man *became* a living being (soul)."[3] From the Jewish perspective, human life is bound up with the survival or resurrection of the body.[4] The evidence of 1 Thessalonians 4:13–5:11 suggests that Paul expected to be alive when Jesus returned. He speaks of "we who are alive and remain" at the time of Jesus' coming. But he has already begun to think of the fate of believers who have died. They will be caught up first to meet the Lord in the air. Only then will "we who are alive and remain" join them. Thus, at this time, Paul thinks of himself as one who would still be alive.

Between the writing of 1 Corinthians and 2 Corinthians Paul came to consider the likelihood of his own mortality, his own death. We can only speculate about what led to this development in his thought.[5]

AGING AND THE IMAGE OF GOD

Where Judaism understood the creation of humans in the image of God to mean that humans could live in a proper relationship with God guided by the Law *(Torah),* Paul saw human relations with God as ruptured. Creation in the *image* of God was, for Paul, an indication of the purpose of God and the potential of human life. The Genesis story, as understood by Paul, is the story of the human failure to fulfil the potential of creation in the *image* of God.[6] Being created in the *image* of God and loved by God, each individual person is of infinite worth, not necessarily for what we are at any given moment, but because of what we may become in God's purpose. That potential is a fundamental ground for our care for all people, especially for the weak who are not able to care for themselves.

We are concerned to develop in ourselves and to nurture the possibility for others, of spiritual growth. That growth is to be found in the realization of the image of God, that is, the potential for *relationship* with God and with others. For Paul, the image of God points to the *completion* of the creation. Alternatively, Paul speaks of the new creation (2 Cor. 5:17 and see Galatians 3:26-28; 6:15).[7] Two questions can be raised at this point: "What is the relevance of the image of God in the life of faith?" and "What about the resurrection?" To these I will return.

We recognize the world as God's creation. This has relevance for the way we live in the world with reverence for life. In this paper we begin with humanity, created in God's image, that is, created for relationship with God and with each other. Spirituality begins with that relatedness to God and each other. The gospel, though it is rooted in the past revelation of God in Christ, is oriented to the future, to the God who is always making all things new, "Behold I make all things new" (Revelation 21:1,5). When we are young we learn to live open to the future. There is no reason why we should ever close our minds to the future if we believe that the future belongs to God, who reveals himself to us as the *alpha* and *omega*, the beginning and the end. This is an important perspective for us to retain as we age.

WE DO NOT LOSE HEART

My Pauline perspective is a reflection on three chapters of *2 Corinthians, chapters 3, 4 and 5*.[8] Taking my cue from Paul: "*Because of this, having this ministry even as we have received mercy, **we do not lose heart**" (2 Corinthians 4:1)

"*Wherefore we do not lose heart, for if our outer person is decaying, our inner person is being renewed day by day*" (4:16).

Thus 4:16 is a resumption of 4:1: "We do not lose heart." The resumption in 4:16 alerts us to the way 4:1 is connected to chapter 3 and 4:16 connects chapter 4 with chapter 5.[9] "Having this ministry, just as we have received mercy, we do not lose heart," we do not get discouraged. The rejection of Paul's ministry and preaching by his own people threatened to discourage him (see 3:1-18, 4:3-4). 2 Corinthians 3-5 deals with Paul's defense of his ministry. But he also addresses the negative and destructive forces that threaten all of our lives in the world. We do not lose heart because we have received mercy (4:1). This rather general description of the basis of our encouragement and positive view of life is spelt out more specifically in the restatement of 4:16 and concerns the effective power of the transforming image of God in the lives of believers. The mercy we have received takes the form that, even though *our outer person is decaying, our inner person is being renewed day by day.* It is not a matter of self-renewal but one of "being renewed," and in a process, "day by day."

Reference to the decay of the outer person is a stark and powerful way to confront us with the aging process. None of us wishes to face the debilitating affects of aging which, in time, make us weak and helpless. We may run from this but there is nowhere to hide from it. How can we face it? For Paul the response is grounded in the experience of God's grace, "As we have received mercy, we do not lose heart." This is an important blessing. It is the blessing of *shalom,* that is a special kind of peace, as we grow older. And yet there is more . . . !

THE TRANSFORMING IMAGE

Paul's specific problem is those who reject his ministry. He argues that the god of this world has blinded the perception of those who do not believe so that they do not see the light of the gospel of the glory of Christ, who is the *image of God.* Paul does not attribute the destructive forces to God. Nor does he say, "What seems to be destructive to us is really God's good purpose." Rather he speaks of the god of this world obstructing the light of the gospel of the glory of Christ, who is the *image of God.* Paul knows, of course, that Genesis teaches that God created humans in the image of God. In spite of this Paul speaks of Christ as the *image* of God in a way that implies that other people, apart from him, are not. Christ is the transforming *imago dei* (see 2 Cor. 3:18) who has the power to make others in the same *image.* This is a process, "from glory to glory" (3:18), "day by day" (4:16).

Here Paul, in tension with Jewish teaching of his time, turns to other accepted Jewish teaching that he creatively uses to make his point. According to Scripture, when Moses looked on God, his own face was temporarily transformed, but the glory faded, it did not last. The believer who beholds the glory of God in the face of Jesus Christ is transformed from glory to glory (3:18; 4:4,6). While the general sense of Paul's argument is clear, the detail is not. The argument of 3:13-18 adopted in this paper can be set out as follows.

1. Moses, whose appearance was temporarily transformed by the glory of God he encountered on the mountain, is contrasted with the appearance of the glory seen in the face of Jesus Christ, the image of God.

2. Although the glory was fading day by day, Moses covered his face and it was hidden from the sons of Israel (see Ex. 34:33, 35). For Paul, the point of contrast is that the face of Moses was veiled from the Israelites whereas believers look on the glory revealed in the face of Jesus Christ with unveiled faces. Paul does not discuss whether the fading glory, reflected from the face of Moses, had the power to transform those who saw. He wished to exploit the metaphor of the veil.

3. The veil over the face of Moses, hiding it from the sons of Israel, now becomes the veil over their *heart* when they read Moses (the law), 3:15. In Hebraic thought, the heart is the centre of moral and spiritual discernment. Thus the law has become veiled from them. They do not discern the message that is hidden there.

4. In contrast, "we" (the believers) with *unveiled face* behold the glory of the Lord and are transformed into *the same image,* 3:18. It is the same image as Christ, who is the image of God, 4:4. The light of the glory of God is to be seen in the face of Jesus Christ, 4:6. Thus we have the powerful metaphor of a face to face *relationship* between the believer and Christ, the image of God.

5. Jesus is seen as the generative *image of God* who has the power to transform others into *the same image,* 3:18. Because the glory of God is seen in the generative *image* of God, Paul uses the participle κατοπτριζόμενοι, a verb used only here in the New Testament. The meaning of this word is obscure. Here it might describe looking at an image as if it were a mirror.[10] The glory seen in this image transforms those who look on it. By looking they reflect the glory of the one who is essentially the image of God. Those who see the glory of God in the face of Jesus Christ *reflect* that glory as they continue to behold it. Because the reflection is continuous (present participle), the glory does not fade and the believer is transformed from glory to glory, day by day.

6. The process of beholding/reflecting the glory of the Lord is clear from the use of the present participle κατοπτριζόμενοι. Beholding is an ongoing process.

7. It is also an inward process because "It is God who said, 'Let light shine out of darkness' who has *shone in our hearts,* with the light of the knowledge of the glory of God in the face of Jesus Christ" (4:4, 6). Just as the veil over the face of Moses becomes a veil over the *heart* of unbelieving Israelites, which is taken away when they turn to the Lord (3:15-16), so believers behold with unveiled faces (3:18) the knowledge of the glory of God in the face of Jesus Christ, 4:6. That is to say, God has caused his light "to shine in our *hearts* with the light of the knowledge of the glory of God in the face of Jesus Christ" 4:6.[11]

8. The inward process of transformation (μεταμορφούμεθα) has been described as a continuing face to face relationship, and as a process of shining in our hearts (3:18; 4:6). It is also described as a process worked by the Spirit. "The Lord is the Spirit; and where the Spirit of the Lord is there is liberty" (3:17). The transformation from glory to glory is "even as by the Spirit of the Lord" (or the Lord, the Spirit) 3:18. See also Romans 5:5 where Paul says that "the love God is poured in our *hearts* by the Holy Spirit who is given to us." Thus God works by means of the Holy Spirit and 2 Cor.3:13-18 suggests that the Spirit works in conjunction with the believing reading of Scripture. In Christ, the veil is taken away, 3:14; for those who turn to the Lord, the veil is taken away, 3:16.

9. The transformation is a process, from glory to glory, day by day 3:18; 4:4, 6, 16.

10. The transforming process of 3:18 is linked to 4:16 by 4:1, 4, 6. Transformation into the image of God involves the paradox that, although our outer being is decaying our inner person is being renewed, day by day, from glory to glory.

Thus, in and through Christ the *potential* of creation in the *image* of God can be realized. This process is a more deeply spiritual and continuing transformation than was experienced by Moses. It does not fade out. Rather it continues as an ongoing process, from glory to glory, day by day, through the agency of the Spirit of the Lord (3:18; 4:6, 16).

"*We* do not lose heart," in spite of the conditions that seem to threaten the transforming power of the gospel in the lives of believers. Paul nowhere softens the harshness of the conditions that we must all face in one way or another in the world. What he does is to stress the rich resource of grace available to enable the believer to struggle through, against all odds. There is a mystery of evil but the central gospel truth is that God is able to and does bring good out of evil (Romans 8:28).

THE PARADOX:
WE HAVE THIS TREASURE IN EARTHEN VESSELS

This paradox is that "We have this treasure in earthen vessels (jars) (ὀστρακίνοιςσκεύεσιν)" (4:7). Paul recognizes the fragility of the human condition, which, at the same time and as a contrast, illuminates the treasure of the transformed life. It shines out more brilliantly from the earthen vessels. This is a brilliant image, both from the context of the Genesis creation story and in the light of modern science. In Genesis God makes humans from the dust of the earth (2:7) and we are told that in death humans return to the ground, "for out of it you were taken; you are dust, and to dust you shall return" (Gen. 3:19). Indeed, the human body can be reduced to a handful of chemicals. Thus Paul recognizes the lowly material composition of human lives.

But Paul does not denigrate the human body in recognizing its earthy origin. The reality of the treasure of the gospel is revealed precisely *in* such human lives. What is amazing is the way frail human lives sustain such hardships and suffering with an amazing strength and endurance. For Paul this shows the way the believer, physically, in the body, participates in the death of Jesus and at the same time manifests the power of his risen life. There is this paradox of the weakness and decay of the body in relation to the transforming power of the risen life announced in Jesus. What is more, this transforming power advances with the growing response to the gospel (4:13-15). But before turning to this theme I want to *re*-emphasize that Paul does not belittle the physical body.

First, I draw your attention to what Paul says in the passage we have just been looking at. "We are always bearing about the *death* of Jesus *in the body* so that the *life* of Jesus may be manifest *in our body*" (4:10). The body, though it is an earthen vessel, is crucial for human life including the life of faith. In the next verse Paul even speaks of the *life* of Jesus being manifest *in our mortal flesh* (4:11).

From the perspective of Pauline spirituality, the body is important. In 1 Cor. 6:12-20 Paul deals with the use and abuse of the body. He concludes by saying, *Do you not know that your body is a temple of the*

Holy Spirit, who is in you, which you have from God, and you are not your own? . . . Glorify God in your body. See also 1 Cor 3:16; 2 Cor 6:16.

Paul also uses the metaphor of the athlete who trains the body to produce maximum performance (1 Cor. 9:24-27). The image of training the body is a crucial strategy in the life of faith because of the importance of the body in the spiritual life. Thus there are grounds for looking after the body as essential to the worship, and service of God. Set this in the context of aging and spirituality and we can say that a sound, healthy, fit body provides a great basis for a vigorous spirituality. Indeed, soundness of body becomes more important the older we grow. Physical fitness has its impact on spirituality.

Nevertheless, Paul's basic point is that we have this treasure in earthen vessels (4:7). The treasure of the gospel shines out of human weakness. It is grace for those who are in need. But weakness is not to be sought for that reason. Paul speaks of an affliction, a thorn in the flesh, a messenger of Satan, from which he earnestly sought relief only to learn that God's answer was, "My grace is sufficient for you" (2 Cor. 12:7-10). Affliction or weakness is not to be sought. But the bearing of affliction is not inconsistent with the gospel. Indeed, the grace of the gospel is a resource in the bearing of affliction. Here, as elsewhere in life, the believer needs to cling to the truth of the gospel, that God is able to, and does bring good out of evil. That does not somehow make the evil good. It demonstrates the grace and power of God to turn all things to the good of those who love and serve him (Romans 8:28). That good depends on the way we respond to evil. It is turned to good for those who love and serve God.

So we come to our resumption, "We do not lose heart." But it is a resumption with a difference. In the hermeneutical circle when we return to the same point we return in a new way because the process has transformed our understanding. We have now a better idea of the forces that threaten to make us lose heart and of the transforming power that Paul affirms can save us from despair.

OUTWARD DECAY AND INWARD RENEWAL

Wherefore we do not lose heart, for even if our outward person is wasting away, our inner person is being renewed day by day (4:16).

First, we notice that Paul speaks of *our outward person* (ὁ ἔξω ἡμῶν ἄνθρωπος) and *our inner [person]* (ὁ ἔξω ἡμῶν). While Paul does not elsewhere speak of the *outward person*,[12] he does use the term *inner person (ἔσω ἄνθρωπον)*in Rom 7.22 [cf. Eph 3:16]. The lack of the specific use of αvΘρωπου" with reference to the inner person in 2 Cor 4:16 is stylistic. It is implied by the use of the term in the first part of the contrast with the *outer person*. This is confirmed by the use of *inner person* Romans 7 [and Eph 3:16]. The use of *inner* implies an outer just as the use of *outer* implies an inner. But what does Paul have in mind?

> Paul nowhere else uses the expression "outer person" but he does write of "our old person" (ὁ παλαιὸς ἡμῶν ἄνθρωπος), Romans 6:6; cf. Colossians 3:9; Ephesians 4:22.

> The expression "our inner [person]" (ὁ ἔσω ἡμῶν [ἄνθρωπος]) is used in Romans 7:22 (τὸν ἔσω ἄνθρωπον).

It seems as if Paul refers to the "new creation" (5:17) in terms of the inner person because its newness is not visible, not fully fashioned and it needs to be renewed day by day. What is visible is the "outer person" which may seem to be unchanged, not a new creation. The outer person is the old person. But a transformation is in process. Thus life in the present is experienced as a struggle, in the tension between the old and the new. How is this to be understood?

First, Paul's use of the expressions "outer person" and "inner person" are not references to the Hellenistic distinction between the mortal body and the immortal soul.[13] The Hellenistic way of reading Paul became attractive in the second century and was given classical expression in the writings of that great neo-Platonist, St. Augustine of Hippo at the end of the third and beginning of the fourth centuries. Paul stands in the Jewish tradition whereby the destruction of the body in death is the destruction of the person. The person does not have a soul but is a living soul (Gen. 2:7). The Hebrew term *nephesh* is translated ψυχή in Greek and often as soul in English. But note Genesis 2:7 does not say *"received* a soul" but *"became* a living soul." Greek dictionaries dealing with the New Testament recognize that ψυχή does not mean soul but is a reference to the self-conscious self. Hope does not lie in the escape of an immortal soul from a mortal body but in God who raises the dead to life, "we know that the one who raised the Lord Jesus will also raise us with Jesus" (4:14). The problem of decay and death is finally dealt with by the resurrection, a new creative act of God, bringing new and transformed life.

Second, nevertheless, the new life is foreshadowed in the renewal of the inner person, day by day (4:16). The resumption of 4:1 reminds us of the connection with 3:18. The ground of encouragement is the transformation of those who, with unveiled faces behold the glory of the Lord (Jesus) and are transformed into his *image,* from glory to glory (3:18, 4:6). Here, the "from glory to glory" corresponds to the "day by day" in 4:16. Paul is talking of a process that begins in this present life. It is a process which deals with the restoration of the *image* (τὴν αὐτὴν εἰκόνα) as believers, beholding the glory of the Lord in the face of Jesus Christ, are transformed (μεταμορφούμεθα) into the same *image* from glory to glory by the Spirit of the Lord. Paul builds on the Genesis notion of humanity created in the *image* of God. But for him the *image* is now found in Jesus alone and in those for whom it is being restored by him. The *image* is not some independent quality which individuals may possess. It involves a mutual relationship with God, established by God and a relationship of servanthood with each other, "and ourselves, your servants for Jesus' sake" (4:5).

Third, the ongoing transformation is the gift of grace and is a ground for hope in the resurrection. It is also the source of the ministry of service because the transforming glory is the light of the gospel of the glory of Christ who is the *image* of God (εἰκὼν τοῦ θεοῦ, 4:4). The response can only be "We do not preach ourselves but Jesus Christ as Lord, and ourselves?–your servants for Jesus' sake" (4:5). Furthermore, the transformation is paradoxical. "We have this treasure in earthen vessels," 4:7 This does not suggest some sort of dualism because the treasure is not separable from the earthen vessels. Yes, and there are cracks in the vessels and they show the marks of wear and tear. The creative light of God has shone in our hearts in the face of Jesus Christ. For Paul this is transforming knowledge even though the earthen vessels remain, cracks and all.

Fourth, only resurrection ultimately deals with decay and death. In the light of eternal glory, faith experiences the renewal day by day and struggles with the momentary afflictions. Faith struggles with the transient visible oppression in the light of the invisible eternal glory. It struggles with the decaying earthly existence in the light of the heavenly new creation where death is swallowed up by life (4:17-5:5). This is the ground of courage (5:6-10). The cracked earthen vessels are the means by which God's grace and glory are present in transforming power in our world.

Fifth and finally, there is continuity between the renewal of the inner person and the resurrection. For Paul this is important. There is a continuity of identity through the transforming process in the present that lays the ground for the risen life. *"He who prepared us for this very thing is God, who has given us* τὸν ἀρραβῶνα *of the Spirit"* (5:5).[14] Aging brings decay. But the renewing grace of God can transform this to reveal God's presence and purpose in remarkable ways. Even here God is able to and does bring good out of evil. And, at the end of the day there is the hope of resurrection.

CONCLUSION:
AGING AND SPIRITUALITY

Aging is something we all face, should we live long enough. Length of life is a blessing from the Lord–this is a biblical perspective expressed again and again in the Old Testament, especially Deuteronomy (4:40; 5:33; 6:2; 11:8-9; 30:20). But it is a mixed blessing because, with age comes decay of physical strength and also of the mind. Yet there is the promise of the renewal of the mind, the renewal of the inner person, day by day even though the cracked and decaying earthen vessel remains. Only resurrection transforms this. In the meantime the challenge is to find those aspects of life which are renewed by the gospel. The restoration of the *image* of God puts the focus on the restored relationship to God for which humans were created and the consequent renewal of relationship with each other. Spirituality involves nurturing relationships in a way that expresses concern for the well being of others, that is an outward view rather than inward looking self-concern. As we grow older we need to struggle to maintain this perspective; it is God's view of things. There is also the challenge to remain open to the newness of the work of God, who is always making all things new. This openness to the new is essential to Christian spirituality. Those of us of older age need this perspective if we are to make an ongoing contribution to the construction of a new and better future *for all of God's creatures.* In this openness we are renewed day by day.

NOTES

1. Paul presupposes the Hebraic understanding of the human person while using the Greek language where the use of body and soul seems to imply a dualism. But for Paul bodily existence is affirmed and thus resurrection is essential to his response to the dilemma of human life in the world. Paul also knows something about stresses

(θλῖψις) on human life in the world including those caused by age and decay. In responding to these he provides insight into our topic today.

2. The reference is to studies carried out in relation to Victoria University in Canada. See David F. Hultsch, Christopher Hertzog, Roger A. Dixon & Brent J. Small, *Memory Change in the Aged* (Cambridge: CUP 1998).

3. It is noteworthy that the 'P' account of humanity created in the image of God (Gen. 1:26-27) has as its counter-part in the 'J' tradition of Gen. 2:7, creation from the dust of the earth and the breath of God to make humans living beings. Each account also deals with the creation of men and women, women being fundamental to creation in the image of God in Genesis 1 but secondary to man in Genesis 2.

4. Unlike some Greek views which saw the body as a limitation from which the soul would escape at death. From the second century onwards the Greek view has been influential in Christianity.

5. It may be that Paul faced a serious life-threatening situation in Ephesus between the writing of 1 and 2 Corinthians.

6. The symbolism of the image of God illuminates the creation of humans with ability to respond in a personal way to God. The ability to respond is the ground of the possibility of a relationship with God. The actualization of this leads to the transformation of believers into the image of Christ, who is the image of God.

7. In 2 Corinthians 5:16-21 Paul asserts that anyone in Christ (the image of God, 4:4) is a new creation (καινήκτίσς), 5:17 and this is a consequence of the ministry of reconciliation which is concerned with the restoration of the alienated to a relationship with God, to a restoration or fulfillment of the image of God (3:18).

8. See for example C.K. Barrett, *The Second Epistle to the Corinthians* (London: A & C Black, 1973); V.P. Furnish, *The Second Epistle to the Corinthian* (New York: The Anchor Bible, Doubleday, 1984).

9. Thus Paul's discussion in 4:1 and 4:16 is part of an exposition of the nature of his ministry in chapters 3-5.

10. Because this verb is used only here in the New Testament it is difficult to be certain of its precise meaning. It certainly means to *behold* the glory of the Lord. This particular verb might have been chosen because it customarily means to behold an image as in a mirror. Here the glory is seen in the face of Jesus Christ who is himself the *image* of God.

11. For the close connection between eyes and heart signaling the understanding of the heart as the organ of moral and spiritual perception see Ephesians 1:18, which speaks of "the eyes of your heart being enlightened."

12. He does use the term ἔξω to refer to outsiders, non-believers.

13. See Stanley Marrow, ΑΘΑΝΑΣΙΑ/ΑΝΑΣΤΑΣΙΣ, "The Road Not Taken," *NTS* 45/4 (1999), 571-86.

14. The expression conveys the sense that the presence of the Spirit is already the beginning of the work that is to be completed in resurrection. It asserts that the beginning is the evidence and assurance of the fullness of life to come in the resurrection.

'Wholeness, Dignity and the Ageing Self': A Conversation Between Philosophy and Theology

Winifred Wing Han Lamb, PhD
Heather Thomson, PhD

This chapter has two sections. The first is written by a philosopher, Winifred Wing Han Lamb; the second by a theologian, Heather Thomson. Their shared interest in theories of the human person brought them into conversation. They describe their approach in the following paragraphs.

SUMMARY. *Winifred Wing Han Lamb:* My philosophical interest straddles the areas of education, religion and theology. As a teacher involved in school philosophy programs, I have also been interested in the philosophy of childhood and particularly in the recurring notion of the 'whole child' in education. In considering what 'wholeness' could mean for children's education, I have also been led to consider what meaning it holds for the self through the 'changing scenes' of life, especially in the face of the challenges of ageing.

Winifred Wing Han Lamb and Heather Thomson, are affiliated with St. Mark's National Theological Centre, School of Theology, Charles Sturt University.

[Haworth co-indexing entry note]: " 'Wholeness , Dignity and the Ageing Self': A Conversation Between Philosophy and Theology." Wing Han Lamb, Winifred, and Heather Thomson. Co-published simultaneously in *Journal of Religious Gerontology* (The Haworth Pastoral Press, an imprint of The Haworth Press, Inc.) Vol. 12, No. 3/4, 2001, pp. 57-76; and: *Aging, Spirituality and Pastoral Care: A Multi-National Perspective* (ed: Elizabeth MacKinlay, James W. Ellor, and Stephen Pickard) The Haworth Pastoral Press, an imprint of The Haworth Press, Inc., 2001, pp. 57-76. Single or multiple copies of this article are available for a fee from The Haworth Document Delivery Service [1-800-342-9678, 9:00 a.m. - 5:00 p.m. (EST). E-mail address: getinfo@haworthpressinc.com].

The notion of 'wholeness' holds an intuitive appeal and invites articulation of the deep truths of our faith with respect to persons in all 'sorts and conditions.' In section one of this chapter, I attempt that articulation. But this conversation needs to be complementary. Our chapter is the beginning of a dialogue between philosophy and theology in which both affirm the ageing self in the light of the human search for wholeness and dignity.

Heather Thomson: My theological research into humanity as an image of God led me to inquire about the way in which we could speak meaningfully of ageing and dying in terms of imaging God. This challenged how God-likeness was to be understood in relation to glory, honour and power, terms associated with imaging God and exerting dominion. In searching for a theological view of the self that would confer dignity on the ageing, I was led into conversation with various philosophies of the self, some very helpful for my task.

It seems to me that, if ageing people are to be counted as having dignity and worth, and not discounted, then one's theory of the human person was significant. In pondering the issue, it appeared that a conversation between philosophy and theology would be fruitful. Hence, this joint paper. We each speak from our own discipline but find resonance with each other's work. We see this as a first step in a constructive conversation. *[Article copies available for a fee from The Haworth Document Delivery Service: 1-800-342-9678. E-mail address: <getinfo@haworthpressinc.com> Website: <http://www.HaworthPress.com> © 2001 by The Haworth Press, Inc. All rights reserved.]*

KEYWORDS. Wholeness, dialogical self, narrative self, continuity, dignity, image of God, the 'loving eye,' sacred power

SECTION ONE–'WHOLENESS' AND THE AGEING SELF

Introduction

In considering the human condition, the theologian Edward Schillebeeckx noted the deep-seated tendency in western thinking to *regard our finitude as a flaw*. He writes:

The basic mistake of many conceptions about creation lies in the fact that finitude is felt to be a flaw, a hurt which as such should not really have been one of the features of the world . . . there is the feeling that . . . mortality, failure, mistakes and ignorance should not be a part of the normal condition of our humanity . . . [1]

This tendency is part of the overall picture of the self in much of traditional theology and philosophy in the west. This is the self that Iris Murdoch describes as follows: . . . this man is with us still, free, independent, lonely, powerful, rational, responsible, brave, the hero of so many novels and books of moral philosophy.[2] Much recent work has been done in re-thinking the self away and apart from these super-human directions. More work still needs to be done especially in relation to the ageing self. Our treatment of dignity and wholeness is part of re-thinking personhood. In the face of ideals such as self-reliance, rational autonomy, self-transparency and confident self mastery, we pose the realities of human loss, fragility, temporality and the experience of inter-subjective dependence. Ours is the beginning of a dialogue between philosophy and theology–between the philosophy of the self and theological anthropology with respect to ageing. On both sides of our dialogue, we each strive to hold to the realities of the human condition on the one hand, while on the other adhering to the biblical promise of wholeness and dignity. This part of the chapter begins with a philosophical discussion of wholeness and what this entails for the ageing self.

Philosophers have identified the vagueness of the notion of 'wholeness' and the popularity of its use in advancing arguments, such as those relating to education. In the debate on the 'whole child' in education, philosophers of education have noted how 'wholeness' is often used as a slogan to advance arguments about educational values.[3] The term is useful for such purposes, not only because it is sufficiently vague but because it also has favorable connotations. It is hard to argue against the slogan that we should educate the 'whole child.'

Although the notion of wholeness is vague and slippery, it does point to some deep intuitions about the value of persons.[4] As we dig a little deeper, we begin to touch on these intuitions. They involve what people are fundamentally like and what our deepest hopes are for them from birth to death.

As claimed earlier, western theology and philosophy have promoted a view of the person as self-reliant, autonomous and rational. Of course, this is not conducive to certain conditions of life in which these qualities are lacking. Childhood is one such condition; old age is another. So, too, are the conditions of disability and illness. It is precisely because of this tension between that view of the self enjoying confident self-mastery and the realities of the human condition, that we pose the crucial question: Are dignity and wholeness possible for the ageing self? My response is arranged in three parts. In exploring the meaning of wholeness, I will look in Parts I and II at various senses of the word in relation to persons. In Part I, I begin by suggesting a few preliminary senses of wholeness and discuss their applicability to the ageing self. While these senses are illuminating, they are insufficient because they give the impression of a static and unchanging self. In Part II, 'Wholeness as continuity and adequacy,' additional senses of 'wholeness' as 'continuity' and 'adequacy' are proposed in which to enlarge our understanding of the ageing self living across time and through change. Part III, 'Wholeness and the Loving Eye,' concludes with the notion of 'wholeness' as *dialogical communion* in which I put forward the idea that wholeness is dependent on others and especially upon their reverence and love in continuing one's own story.

In looking at the different senses of 'wholeness,' my purpose is to go beyond semantics. I want somehow to show that at the conceptual level, the notion of wholeness encourages us to think about the self in a certain way. It needs to be affirmed in more human directions while being theologically grounded in the doctrine of the human person as made in the image of God. With this kind of foundation, my purpose is to see how a philosophy of the self can help us to think affirmatively about the ageing self.

Part I. 'Wholeness as Comprehensiveness, Integration, Coherence and Intactness'

The first two senses of 'wholeness' are 'comprehensiveness' and 'integration.'[5] 'Comprehensiveness' suggests 'balance' and 'breadth.' This reference is most applicable in cases where, for example, we refer to the education of 'the whole person.' Here we mean education that addresses *all aspects* of a person. 'Integration,' on the other hand, opposes wholeness to fragmentation, unboundedness and confusion. But what do these words mean in relation to persons? The sense of wholeness as 'integration' is more pertinent to our interest in suggesting 'coherence' and 'internal harmony.' 'Integration,' 'coherence' and 'internal harmony' are states in which the person is able to order their conflicting desires and priorities and act in a way consistent with their values and goals. This may be contrasted with the person in whom there is no such order or hierarchy of desires. The philosopher Joel Feinberg provides a graphic description of such a person who is 'a battlefield for all his constituent elements, tugged this way and that and fragmented hopelessly.' Such a person is incapable of exercising autonomous choice being 'tied in knots by the strands of his own wants.'[6]

It is, of course, a mark of maturity to have sufficient self-knowledge and self-mastery to arrive at such internal coherence and integration. One of the things that we desire as we age is the sense of peace and poise (in a way) that comes from having reckoned with our deepest conflicts so that we no longer contend with a 'traffic jam' of desires. In addition to this source of coherence and inner tranquillity is the peace that comes from the deep acceptance of our finitude and of the opportunities we have enjoyed in our lifetime. This kind of acceptance is vital for the nurturing of inter-generational relationships. To be in a position to encourage the young, give them our blessing for what they do, graciously 'step down' from responsibilities of various kinds, requires that such inner conflicts be understood and reconciled. This kind of wholeness naturally requires not only self-understanding, but also a good deal of personal work.

'Intactness' continues the idea of such personal work and such self-cultivation. It is a kind of 'boundedness' in which one's identity is preserved through a proper appreciation of boundaries, between private and public domains of life, with a proper framework of hope to interpret and hold our experiences.

We are reminded of times we have to pull ourselves together when we are confused and 'thrown.' In some moments, intactness, integration and coherence is an achievement of the self. However, we also know from experience that this achievement is also highly dependent upon others. The courage we possess depends to a large extent on what we have received from them. So, too, does our self-esteem.

However, the dominant view of the self in western philosophy has not sufficiently acknowledged the dimension of *self-in-relation* and of the ways in which our identity depends upon the recognition of others. The philosopher Charles Taylor asserts that modern western thinking has been 'overwhelmingly monological' in character because it advances a view of the self as a self sufficient 'thing.' Or, in philosophical language, a 'substance' that is intact and entire on its own. In contrast to this view of the self as atomistic substance, Taylor says that our identity crucially depends on our relations with others. He contends:

We become full human agents, capable of understanding ourselves, and hence of defining our identity, through our acquisition of rich human 'languages' of art, of gesture, of love. . . . We define our identity always in dialogue with, sometimes in struggle against, the things our significant others want to see in us. Even after we outgrow some of these others–our parents, for instance–and they disappear from our lives, the conversation with them continues within us as long as we live.[7]

Taylor explains how this kind of understanding of personal identity gives rise to a new acknowledgement of the importance of *recognition* and of how we are regarded by others. In this way, Taylor rejects the monological self in favor of the *dialogical self,* i.e., the self-formed in relation.

The relevance of this to children and to the growing years is obvious. We now know a good deal about self-fulfilling prophecies with respect to the development of the young; how recognition of a positive nature encourages success in every way. How others 'know' me is not a neutral thing nor does it not have neutral implications. Others can know me in a gentle, hopeful and loving way in which what they convey to me about myself is based upon true facts, well founded judgements and, if they are realists, no illusions either. But included in that knowledge is *hope:* the expectation that I will learn, that I will see more clearly; and, that I will work out the difficulties I face. In contrast to this generous knowledge is the claim of one to know all about me, to possess the standpoint to 'sum me up.' When this also includes the all-knowing prophecy that certain imperfections and faults and incapacities will *always* be there and never be overcome, I am colonized and totalized by this knowing. 'What do you expect? She's hopeless!' will be re-played at various points in my life. The relevance of this to childhood is obvious. But the aged, too, depend upon how they are known.[8] In the later years, recognition and dialogical relations assume a new poignancy. I will return to this insight.

Part II. 'Wholeness as Continuity and Adequacy'

The recognition that is given to us by 'loving knowledge' is one that is based on unconditionality. Loving knowledge does not just see the negatives in such a way that these define the person. Rather, because love hopes all things, those who love us will also see us moving on. The comments: 'she'll be fine'; 'she'll learn in due course'; and, 'she'll find her way' convey loving knowledge borne of hope. Such a judgement is not based solely on what the person has done but on *the imagination of possibilities.* In theological language, such unconditionality is called *grace.* Moltmann defines grace as 'demonstrative value of being'[9]; a person is unconditionally acceptable regardless of what they do or accomplish. Someone has intrinsic worth and they do not have to prove anything to be loved. There emerges here another sense of wholeness as 'adequacy.' The enjoyment of this kind of wholeness is a gift from others. In this enjoyment, one feels unconditionally accepted and entirely 'adequate.' Such a state leads not only to joy but also to creativity because the individual is free to know and to explore the world in which she has found a home. Moltmann calls this 'productive play.'

The idea of play and of a person reaching out in creativity reminds us that the self is active. Indeed, it is active in many directions. One direction in the later years is its movement backwards and forwards in memory and in the construction and re-negotiation of memory. The more static notions of "integration," "coherence" and "intactness" do not convey this movement in the self. To convey the temporal and active sense we need to think of wholeness as a kind of "continuity." J.M. Heaton describes this as *'the thread that joins us to our infancy*[10]. It is a continuity maintained and re-negotiated throughout life. Continuity is part of our self-narrative that flows creatively when there is growth. However, it is disjunctively broken at times of trauma and crises. Wholeness as continuity could be understood as the way of keeping the self-narrative alive and developing in a way that is commensurate with experience and understanding. The later years offer a good opportunity for wisdom and a sense of perspective in understanding life as part of the construction of a life narrative. Such a story of one's life could be a way of reckoning with conflicts considered in Part I. This will include both conflicts and regrets about things done badly or not at all. The notion of 'continuity' picks up this task of reckoning with one's life with events and achievements that are a cause of celebration, but also with all the discontinuities, randomness and waste that form the stuff of most human lives. 'Continuity' is an active notion of wholeness that shows the healthy resilience of the self to embrace both the positive and the negative. It encompasses tragedy and hope.[11]

The task of achieving continuity of the self is therefore an active one that involves re-negotiating memories, values and life goals. When this is done in the light of grace, hope and eternity, there can be rejoicing and forgiveness. The philosopher Søren Kierkegaard said that living in the light of eternity involves continuous growth towards 'purity of heart.'[12]

For him 'purity of heart' includes 'slowly and honestly' facing up to one's life and life narrative in such a way that involves a process of self-unification and overall 'sense.' So, in Kierkegaard's notion of 'purity of heart,' we see how 'integration' is achieved in the light of the temporal 'continuity' of a person's life.

Old age brings insight and wisdom in that undertaking. It affords both time and perspective. However, it can also bring the abrupt loss of continuity. If, as Taylor says, the self is dialogically made with and against many other people in our lives and if our "conversation" with them continues within us as long as we live, what happens if conversation cannot be continued?

Part III. 'Wholeness and the Loving Eye'[13]

Grandpa's Biscuits[14]

> At South Granville Retirement Home
> wrinkles are admitted quite
> openly, if noticed at all.
> A flurry of branches is observable
> through a window.
> Grandpa likes the view.
> He wonders why he cannot
> see it at night time.
> He often has the curtains
> open in the afternoon
> to allow the sun set to put
> him to sleep
> with its pink half light
> blushing on his wrinkled cheeks.
> It seems to please the
> tired sun to drowse
> upon his face.
> He says things that nobody knows the
> meaning of, as if reason had
> let him go,
> and that was his pension.
> He always remembers to let
> you go first through a doorway
> or sitting down,
> but he can't (for the

life of him) remember how the buttons go on
his shirt. "Go ahead," he says and motions
to the door,
letting the buttons slip.
Grandpa had become the
dry husk of the person he had always
been: he does all the things that
he has done all his life,
but without the reasons.

There are lines in his skin,
there's a spot on his forehead,
his hair is grey and white.
His eyes are sometimes red.
His hands clutch their histories–
or a crumbling digestive biscuit
which always has a bite taken out of it,
but rarely any more than that.
Come to think of it,
I don't think I've
ever seen him finish one.
Occasionally,
when looking around his room
at all the things–
the shoe horns, the hats,
the photographs of relatives
that he no longer recognises–
you will find a forgotten,
half-eaten biscuit
forming a puddle of crumbs
where it sits.
All attention is on the present
biscuit, and if that one was lost
he gets another from the tin
beside his bed.
The irregular, inimitable,
unrepeatable bite marks
stretch out like tiny
headlands into space,
whilst the air laps round
in waves

persuading the crumbs from the precipice.
Whether they came
directly off the biscuit or from
the wrinkly edges of his mouth,
the crumbs would always
find their way to
the ground. And it never mattered.

In fact, it was good.
They say that God took
seven days to make the world. It was
as if, after eighty years in that
world, Grandpa had decided that it needed
a new floor.
And that floor was being
made with the silence
and subtlety of dew
dripping amongst the grass.
You hardly noticed.
You hardly noticed that
a life was crumbling in front
of you because it was doing so
without protest,
without tragedy or
without complaint,
but with the quietness and humility
of a dry biscuit becoming
the air.

Most of the phone
calls we have got at three o'clock in
the morning have been accidents.
There is one coming that won't be.
But, although the biscuit tin would be empty,
I'm sure there'll be a half-eaten one,
lurking secretively in that room,
amongst the shoe-horns,
beside a lost watch,
or maybe making dust behind a photo of Grandma.

In the rooms and down the
corridors, Grandpa's peers
are learning how to walk again.
Because, you know,
after eighty or so years of walking
  without thinking,
  you tend
  to forget
  which foot
  goes
  first.

by Julian Lamb, Canberra

Printed with permission from *St. Mark's Review*, No. 182, Winter 2000

The poem 'Grandpa's Biscuits' describes Albert (my own father) who had a full and rich life and whose gentlemanly behavior stayed intact through the loss of memory and the ability to function in other ways. Albert talks because, as always, he relishes a conversation. In my experience of speaking with him, I still enjoy his use of language with its rich and idiosyncratic vocabulary. I also enjoy over-hearing conversations he has with friends similarly afflicted. (Not ever having been a good listener, I even wonder if my father is enjoying more mutuality now that he has lost the sense of the precise meanings of words!) In such exchanges on the third floor of South Granville Lodge, I hear the natural rhythms and cadences of a conversation, as well as the liveliness and mutuality that make conversations nourishment for us. Perhaps communication isn't everything after all. Perhaps communion is deeper still.

Albert has lost the ability to re-construct his self-narrative and to re-visit his memories in a way that we can share. He is vulnerable to how others now construct him. He is vulnerable to being colonized by totalizing knowledge of relatives and friends and careers. If they regard him as demented, annoying, totally uninteresting and just a 'poor thing,' or 'that gentleman with the nice smile,' he will become that for them. However, his sense of continuity can be embraced by the loving knowledge of another in a spirit of unconditionality. In the poem 'Grandpa's Biscuits,'[15] Albert's grandson, Julian takes up the loving task of continuity. The self continues to be made dialogically, even when it is no longer the agent of its own self construction.

But continuity doesn't happen in one direction, it is not simply a monologue. By this I mean that Julian is not the sole agent of construction here. Through the loving gaze, he is also constructing the thread of his own life in the light of the possible loss of features that many see as essential to the self and to its dignity and wholeness. The relationship in this poem illustrates dialogical communion in which wholeness is achieved not through agency and strength of the obvious kind but through love and the mutual appreciation of our finitude and *the demonstrative value of our being*.

In the second half of this essay, Heather Thomson develops the idea of the dialogical formation of the self as a power (again, not of the obvious kind) conferred on us to reflect glory and honour as bearers of God's image. She reminds us of our inescapable mutuality in the assertion that we have the 'awe-ful' power to give honour to others and to 'call into being,' or alternatively, to diminish and thwart life in them.[16] This reminds us again that wholeness, like dignity, while intrinsic to human beings, is also vulnerable to loss and requires mutuality and responsibility to realise.

Of course, from the Christian point of view, the stories of our lives cannot be fully told this side of the *eschaton*. But they must nevertheless be told. This account is redemptive if the story of a life is told with love, in openness, to both the brokenness and discontinuities of the human condition, and also to all the possibilities of God's grace. Eschatologically, the notion of wholeness as 'continuity' takes on further meaning because from the perspective of eternal life we think of this life as continuing in a *'new kind of temporality into which the whole diachronic extent of a person's life is in some way taken through healing and transformation.'*[17] However, this direction of enquiry deserves another discussion on its own!

SECTION TWO–DIGNITY AND THE AGEING SELF

This section addresses the question of dignity and wholeness in the ageing self through the tradition of Christian theology. Central to a Christian understanding of the dignity of the human person is the belief that humanity was made in the image and likeness of God. It must be admitted, however, that few theologians take the ageing self into account when discussing the image of God. In fact, if we turn our attention to the frail aged, those who are wheelchair-bound or bed-ridden and in full-time care, those who have lost their powers of speech, sight, hearing, lost their mobility, memory or continence, such people do not fit easily into traditional theology concerning the image of God. Let me give you three examples.

First, according to the creation theology of Genesis 1, humanity was not only made to the image and likeness of God but was also given dominion over the earth. Theologians differ as to how closely the dominion given to humanity is a result of their being in the image of God, or is something independent. Nevertheless, there remains a connection in this text between imaging God and having dominion. Both confer on humanity authority and power. Further, in reflecting on the wonders of creation and the place of human beings within it, Psalm 8 speaks of humanity as 'little less than God, crowned with glory and honour.' This psalm of praise and wonder goes on to say, 'You have given them dominion over the works of your hands; you have put all things under their feet.'

These texts seem to assume adults in the prime of their lives, confident masters and mistresses of their domain. Being in the image of God and having dominion are associated with glory, honour and power. But what of the person who has lost dominion over his or her own body, let alone the power to care for the earth and all that is in it? Where is the glory and honour in one who is wheelchair-bound, who has nothing under their feet besides a pair of old slippers? To include the frail aged in the notion of the image of God is to re-think glory, honour and power, as well as the way in which the image is applied to humanity.

The second example concerns the definitions of the image. What counts as being God-like, and what is not counted? Although we may be created in the image and likeness of God, it is clear from scripture and from reason that we are not ourselves divine. We are not God. And one significant difference is that human beings age and die. In what way, then, are we God-like?

The early church writers came to conclude that the image of God referred to our souls, our minds, or our inner person. It is in a spiritual sense that we reflect God, or at least we have the capacity to do so, should we choose the right things to do and to love. In this understanding, it is the *body* that is *not* in God's image. The human body is a sign of our mortality, and how can this be a reflection of the immortal God?

Augustine made this point clearly. His emphasis on creation 'out of nothing' was to ensure that what was created was something new. It was not somehow an extension of God. Humanity, and the rest of creation, is not God, nor are we consubstantial or co-eternal with God.[18] Even our souls or spirits were created and are not to be thought of as the same substance as God. Nevertheless, Augustine argues that it is only in the soul that we bear the image of God. 'Who,' he asks, 'would be so utterly out of his mind as to say that we are or shall be similar to God in the body? In the inner [person] therefore is this likeness.'[19]

Is the ageing and dying body, then, a reminder of dissimilarity to God? In what way may the concept of God-likeness incorporate the physical body?

The third example concerns the New Testament teaching from Paul that Christ is the true image of God, and we are made anew to the image God as we are conformed to Christ (Col. 1:15; Eph. 4:22-24; Rom. 8:29; 2 Cor. 3:18; 2 Cor. 4:4; Heb. 1:3). If this teaching is reduced to seeing Christ as our example of God-likeness (the one for us to imitate), we will find that we have no example in Christ as to how to live well into old age. There is much to be said on Christ as image of God. At first glance, however, ageing is not one of them.

From these three examples it can be shown that the traditional doctrine of the image of God does not directly and obviously address the dignity of the ageing self. I propose to reconsider the points made above to show how Christian teaching concerning humanity and the image of God confers on the aged a dignity and worth that requires our honour and respect. First, I will address the creation account in Genesis 1 and reconsider the notions of dominion, glory, honour and power. Second, I will revisit Christ as image of God. Here I will propose an iconic view of the image as icon, and ask what place the body and flesh has in this. Third, I will consider our imaging of God in terms of God as Trinity. I hope here to incorporate being cared for, suffering, dying as being God-like.

Let us first return to the Genesis text. It is generally agreed by biblical scholars that this text was written during the time when the Jewish people were exiled in Babylon, wondering what went wrong, where they had come from, and how they might return to their homeland. Their minds were cast back to their origins and to their relation to God in this genesis. In conceiving there that all human beings were made to the image and likeness of God, the writer of Genesis 1 was attempting to give expression to an impression that there is something sacred and of value about each human being as human, which historical circumstances cannot take away. Nor can geographical place, or one's position in society or one's achievements add to or take away from human worth.

The Jewish people in exile appeared to be no-bodies, worthless, and knew themselves to be the losers historically. Yet, the writer of Genesis 1 used poetic language to aim at a reality more real than appearances.[20]

To call human beings the image of God is not descriptive language. It is rather a proclamation. It is an address to us from outside of ourselves. In this sense we are reminded that we are not self-made or self-determined. Rather, the dignity of our being is grounded in a word prior to any human word or action. If God regards us with a loving eye and establishes our being as a reflection of God, who are we to do otherwise? This point is important if all, including young children and the elderly, are to be given the dignity and worth that is their due.

Some of the early church writers attempted to express this using metaphorical language. For example, the image was likened to an imprint on a coin.[21] We are stamped with a worth that no-one and nothing can take away. Adding to this metaphor, we can say that a coin does not lose its value if dropped in the gutter or trodden into the dirt. So, too, if through historical circumstance, bad fortune or bad decisions on our part, we find ourselves in the gutter or trodden into the dirt, we do not lose our worth. Nor do we do so as we age and die.

Another metaphor comes from Clement of Alexandria. He suggested that the image is like a love-charm. It is something given to us which ties us to God, and makes us dear to God for our own sake.[22]

But what of dominion, glory, honour and power? We need to keep in mind that dominion is given to humanity as a whole. We are not each held responsible for all things all of the time. Dominion, in terms of care for each other and for the earth, contains within it the assumption that we grow into this responsibility and will grow out of it as individuals. However, as a human race and in human societies, we will continue to be called towards this task, honour and responsibility.

In what, then, does our glory and honour consist? It is easy to associate glory with our achievements, with the adulation of others, with being better than others, with recognition of our worthiness compared with other people. Yet this sense of glory is not to be found even in the text of Psalm 8. The glory there is in relation to the other animals of the earth, and to God, not in relation to other humans. Nor does the life and teaching and death of Christ allow for a glory that seeks the attention and envy of other people. Rather he renounces, denounces and undermines such assumptions. Our glory can only be founded on a humble acceptance of our being which was made with a special status a little less than God. This is a gift to be received and honored.

This leads inevitably to a reflection on power. A number of contemporary theologians have alerted me to the connection between the power of God in calling us into being and the power we have in relation to each other to do the same. Beverly Harrison refers to the 'awe-ful and awe-some truth that we have the power, through acts of love or lovelessness literally to create one another.' She says that if our power-in-relation to each other is God-like then we will act each other into well-being. If we misuse our sacred power, we 'thwart life and maim each other.'[23] If we are to live as human beings corresponding to God, then we will live righteously, that is, in right relations, giving each person their due. As Eberhard Jungel puts it:

Those who live out of the righteousness of God will . . . respect the other person as one irrevocably accepted by God, prior to all possible achievements and successes, and in spite of all actual failures and defeats.[24]

Jungel sees this as a fundamental challenge to an achievement-oriented society. It challenges the status we give to those people who can do little or nothing for their own existence–young children, the sick, the handicapped and disabled and the elderly. If we are to live righteously, we will give each person their due, and we cannot escape the power we have in relation to each other in this regard. We can only ask how that power is being used–in a God-like manner to maintain others in well-being, or demonically to diminish and distort the being of others?

We turn now to our second question. What may we learn about dignity and the ageing self from a consideration of Christ as image of God? There is more mystery and depth here than can be reasonably explored within the constraints of available text. There are however a few brief reflections than can be made.

The first concerns the word 'image' which is a translation of the Greek word 'icon.' An icon is something that refers beyond itself to God. It is a window that is seen through rather than a picture that is looked at. To refer to humanity as the image of God is to say that we have a significance that points beyond ourselves. To call Christ the true image of God is to say that he, more than any other, is a window onto God, revealing God's love, forgiveness, mercy, healing and reconciliation, through his life for us. Further, he is icon for us, in and through his body, not in spite of it.

What difference does this make to dignity and older persons? It means that the body can be incorporated into the image of God, as an icon that refers beyond itself. Although St Augustine did not count the body as being in God's image, he did consider that God communicates with us in and through the flesh. And God's fullest word to us, of grace and truth, was through the physical body of Jesus Christ, the Word made flesh. Augustine did not quite resolve the dilemma between a dualistic and a unified view of the human person. I would argue for the unified view. It is in and through our bodies that we show love or withhold love, that we reach out in reconciliation or turn our backs. It is as a unified self, body and soul, that we are windows onto God. Still, what of the aged person who is bed-ridden and unable to be active in any way? How might they yet be considered as an icon of God? Two answers can be proposed.

On the one hand, an aged and dying person may appear little more than a bag of bones. Yet their very bones are a window on a life lived, from the day they were somebody's newborn baby. Unless we can keep alive a narrative view of human life and situate people in the many stories to which they have belonged and continue to belong, society may reduce people to a particular 'present' time and fail to understand them in the fullness of their lives. *How* their lives may have given glimpses of God is a matter for God, and those who knew them well, to answer. The importance of a narrative view of the self is a point that Winifred Lamb has also made.

On the other hand, frail aged people may be considered as icons of Christ in the following way. Although it is true that Jesus never grew old and we cannot imitate Jesus as an elderly person, it *is* true that he did suffer and die. His suffering was not only of physical pain but of ignobility and humiliation, experiences shared by those who lose their capacities and powers in increasing old age. There is much in his story with which the elderly can identify with and be consoled by. In taking on mortal flesh, God identifies with our experiences of humiliation and mortality, and makes them God's own.

This leads to a third and final point. If, in Christian theology, our being in the image of God confers the fundamental dignity of human beings on us, what difference does it make that God is Trinity? How do we image God as Trinity?

This question is not new. St Augustine developed a Trinitarian view of the image of God. He located the image in the rational mind and argued that, just as God is a unity of being and a trinity of relations, so too are our minds a unity in themselves. But they are also a trinity of relations between the memory, the understanding and the will.

More recent scholarship has shifted the location of the Trinitarian image. Instead of being seen to be within each individual, it has been relocated among us, in human relations. That is, humanity images the

Trinitarian God in so far as we relate to each other with the mutual respect and equality that is the hallmark of the relations within the trinity. Karl Barth argued along these lines and contemporary feminist theologians are doing the same.[25] Catherine LaCugna, for example, suggests that Augustine's view of the Trinitarian image was somewhat abstract, and 'contributed to the idea of the self as an "individual" rather than . . . as someone who comes to self through another.'[26] She wishes to relocate the Trinitarian image among us, in the communion we have with one another, reflecting the communion among persons in the trinity.

In relation to the ageing self, some implications of this Trinitarian theology of the image can be readily drawn out. I have discussed already our sacred power in relation to each other, and this Trinitarian theology reinforces what was said earlier. However, I would argue that when we think about being God-like in relation to each other, we tend to think of ourselves as active agents, offering care, healing the sick, releasing the captives, and so forth. I would like to incorporate into our understanding of God, that God is also one who, in Christ, received care. He was himself held and nurtured as a small child, was fed and sheltered by others, was anointed with perfume before his passion, and when he died his body was lovingly taken down from the cross by his friends and family, and prepared for burial.

The point is that both caring and being cared for can be understood to be God-like. We need not feel humiliated when, as we age, we become dependent and need care. God in Christ has incorporated the giving and receiving of care into the life of God.

So, too, with suffering and death. As Christ suffered and died, suffering and dying need not be seen as foreign to God. These can count as being God-like. But we need to exercise caution. Some suffering and some deaths ought to be the subject of protest while some need to be accepted as part of our natural lives as mortal, finite creatures. We cannot easily compare a death from old age with the death of Christ. However, my point is that death itself need not be counted as foreign to God or as something that separates us from the love of God, or that it even counts us out of being in the image of God. Consideration of God as Trinity, particularly of the humanity of God in Christ, is arguably important for understanding the dignity of the ageing self.

This chapter has approached the topic of 'Dignity, wholeness and the ageing self' from insights gained through the disciplines of philosophy and theology. In some theories of the human person, the aged remain barely human. They are a mere shadow of what it means to be a human being. We have argued for an anthropology that allows the ageing self to be given dignity and worth. We have done this in the following ways.

First, we have advocated a shift away from a view of the self as autonomous and self-determined to one that is relational. That is not only to say that we *have* relationships, but that we are each constituted in and through our relationships. In philosophical terms this has been referred to as the 'dialogical self,' and in theological terms it is our 'sacred power' in relation to each other. Second, we have argued for a shift away from any static notions of the self, which are timeless and ahistorical, to a narrative view of the self, where a person is situated in all the stories that make up their lives. The poem "Grandpa's Biscuits" is an example of the way in which the story of Albert's life is honored and continued on in the poetry of his grandson. Finally, we have both spoken on the power of love in bringing each other into, and maintaining each other in, well-being.

One can only hope that these initial reflections might form a basis on which further thinking may fruitfully emerge on the dignity, worth and wholeness of the ageing person.

NOTES

1. Quoted in Fergus Kerr, *Theology After Wittgenstein* (Oxford: Blackwell, 1986), 184.

2. Quoted in ibid., 5.

3. See Ron Best, ed., *Education, Spirituality and the Whole Child* (London: Cassell, 1996); see also Peter Standish, "Postmodernism and the education of the whole person," *Journal of Philosophy of Education* 29 (1) (1995): 121-35; Winifred Wing Han Lamb, "Philosophy for Children and the 'Whole Child'," *Critical and Creative Thinking* 8 (1) (2000).

4. See T.H. McLaughlin, "Education of the Whole Child?" in Ron Best, ed., ibid., 9.

5. Ibid, 12.

6. Joel Feinberg, "The Idea of a Free Man," in *Educational Judgements Papers in the philosophy of education* edited by James F. Doyle (London & Boston: Routledge and Kegan Paul, 1973), 149.

7. Charles Taylor, "The Politics of Recognition," in *Multiculturalism-Examining the Politics of Recognition* edited by Amy Gutman (Princeton, NJ: Princeton University Press, 1994), 25-73.

8. Philosopher Lorraine Code is illuminating on the danger of colonizing through knowledge. She writes, "Where there is a difference in power, knowledge, expertise, a claim that "I know just how you feel" can readily expand into a claim that I will tell you how you feel, and/will be right, even though you might describe them differently, for your perceptions are ill-informed, and my greater expertise must override them." The relevance of this to the care of the elderly is obvious. See "I Know Just How You Feel:

Empathy and the Problem of Epistemic Authority," in Lorraine Code, *Rhetorical Spaces: Essays on Gendered Locations* (New York: Routledge, 1995), 130.

9. Jurgen Moltmann, *Theology and Joy* (London: SCM Press, 1967), 43.

10. J.M. Heaton, "Ontology and Play," in *Phenomenology and Education,* edited by B. Curtis & Wolfe Mays (London: Metheun, 1978), 124.

11. The philosopher Paul Ricoeur drew a distinction between two kinds of identity *idem* (which emphasizes ontological sameness, or permanence over time) and *ipse* (which captures the idea of personal identity through self-continuity). See Paul Ricoeur, *Oneself as Another* (Eng. Chicago: Chicago University Press, 1992. The theologian Kevin Vanhoozer says that as ways of understanding the self's identity through time, the heart of the difference between *idem* and *ipse* identity is the question of temporality. The two notions of identity reflect the attempt either to escape from temporality, or to trust in its ultimate meaningfulness. The idea of "continuity" expresses *ipse* identity, an identity *through time*. See Kevin J. Vanhoozer, *The Trinity in a Pluralistic Age–Theological Essays on Culture and Religion* (Michigan & Cambridge, UK: Eerdmanns Grand Rapids, 1997), 46-7.

12. S. Kierkegaard, *Purity of Heart is to will one thing,* trans. Douglas V. Steere (New York: Harper, 1956).

13. This is Sally McFague's phrase, see McFague, *Super, Natural Christians: How We Should Love Nature* (Minneapolis, Minnesota: Fortress Press, 1997), 35.

14. I am grateful to Julian for allowing me to refer to his poem. It is re-printed through kind permission of *St Mark's Review.*

15. See end of section.

16. See Thomson's reference to Beverly Harrison on p. 72

17. See the discussion on the images of the resurrection and new creation in Richard Bauckham & Trevor Hart, *Hope Against Hope-Christian Eschatology in Contemporary Context* (London: Darton Longman & Todd (Trinity & Truth Series), 1999), 126-32.

18. Augustine, *On Genesis Against the Manichees,* 6. 10; 7. 11.

19. Augustine, *Letters,* XCII, 3.

20. P. Ricoeur, *Interpretation Theory: Discourse and the Surplus of Meaning* (Texas: Christian University, Fort Worth, 1976), 67.

21. Clement of Alexandria, *The Stromata,* VII. iii; Origen, *Treatise on Prayer,* XXII. 4; Gregory of Nyssa, *On the Making of Man,* XVI. 13 and *Sermon on the Sixth Beatitude*; Augustine, *The Trinity,* XII. 3. 16.

22. Clement of Alexandria, *The Instructor,* I. iii.

23. B. Harrison, "The power of anger in the work of love," in *Feminist Theology: A Reader,* edited by A. Loades (London: SPCK, 1990), 203.

24. E. Jungel, "Living out of righteousness," in *Theological Essays II,* edited by J.B. Webster, T. & T. Clark (Edinburgh, 1995), 256.

25. E.A. Johnson, *She Who Is: The mystery of God in feminist theological discourse* (New York: Crossroads, 1994), 223; C.M. LaCugna, ed., *Freeing Theology: The essentials of theology in feminist perspective* (San Francisco: Harper, 1993), 88-89.

26. LaCugna, *Freeing Theology,* 89.

The Getting and Losing Wisdom

Don Thomson, PhD

He that is not handsome at twenty, nor strong at thirty, nor rich at forty, nor wise at fifty, will never be handsome, strong, rich, or wise (G.H) No man is born wise (17th century)

SUMMARY. The role of aging and culture in the attainment of wisdom is examined in this chapter. The concept of wisdom in industrialised societies is briefly explored. It is argued that both biology and culture can be positive or negative factors in the capacity of a person to be "wise." It is concluded that, for many, the negative impact of biological factors of aging are overwhelming, but, for a few, aging enriches their insight. *[Article copies available for a fee from The Haworth Document Delivery Service: 1-800-342-9678. E-mail address: <getinfo@haworthpressinc.com> Website: <http://www.HaworthPress.com> © 2001 by The Haworth Press, Inc. All rights reserved.]*

KEYWORDS. Wisdom, aging, expertise, cultural aging, biological aging

Aging conjures up conflicting images. On the one hand aging has, through the centuries, being linked to wisdom, on the other hand, since ancient times there has been a wide-spread perception that an inevitable

---

Don Thomson is Professor of Psychology, Charles Sturt University, Bathurst, Australia, and has researched memory and related issues for over 30 years.

[Haworth co-indexing entry note]: "The Getting and Losing Wisdom." Thomson, Don. Co-published simultaneously in *Journal of Religious Gerontology* (The Haworth Pastoral Press, an imprint of The Haworth Press, Inc.) Vol. 12, No. 3/4, 2001, pp. 77-88; and: *Aging, Spirituality and Pastoral Care: A Multi-National Perspective* (ed: Elizabeth MacKinlay, James W. Ellor, and Stephen Pickard) The Haworth Pastoral Press, an imprint of The Haworth Press, Inc., 2001, pp. 77-88. Single or multiple copies of this article are available for a fee from The Haworth Document Delivery Service [1-800-342-9678, 9:00 a.m. - 5:00 p.m. (EST). E-mail address: getinfo@haworthpressinc.com].

consequence of aging is decline and incompetency. That such diametrically opposed views of aging co-exist raises the possibility that there is an element of truth to both positions, namely, that with age, some people become wise, whereas other people lose their intellectual capacity and their insight. In this chapter I will be exploring why it is that these two contradictory views on aging have wide currency. To this end, I will first discuss what it might mean for someone to be said to be wise and how age and wisdom might be related. A number of studies which have examined attributes of wisdom as a function of age will be then reviewed. The thesis of this chapter is that wisdom is not a unidimensional concept, and like beauty, is in the eye of the beholder. Whether experience, knowledge, or skills of an older person are perceived as wisdom may depend on how much that experience, knowledge, and skills contribute to the goals of the community in which the older person resides. Thus, in large measure, the status of older persons in the community and how wisdom is defined are likely to be correlated.

CONCEPTUALIZING WISDOM

Wisdom, according to the Shorter Oxford English Dictionary is "the capacity of judging rightly in matters relating to life and conduct; soundness of judgement in the choice of means and ends." While few would quibble with this definition, it provides little insight as to how that capacity is to be assessed, and what constitutes "judging rightly" and how "soundness of judgement" is determined. Thus, the decision as to whether a person has judged "rightly" made a "sound" decision must invariably be made retrospectively and not prospectively, and made on the basis of the values of the decision-maker. Freeman[1] and Chandler and Holiday[2] have made a similar observation.

Nor does the dictionary definition indicate what the characteristics of wise persons are. The question of what characteristics wise persons possess will depend on how a particular culture operationally defines wisdom. Baltes and his associates[3] and other writers[4] have attempted to sketch out defining characteristics of a wise person. However, the different writers appear to conceptualise wisdom in very different ways, although the differences may be more apparent than real, and reflect emphasis rather than structural differences.

According to Holiday and Chandler[5] a wise person possesses five attributes, exceptional understanding, judgment and communication skills, general competence, interpersonal skills, and social unobtrusiveness.

These five attributes can be encompassed within three categories or types of knowledge: general competence, experienced-based pragmatic knowledge, and reflective skills. General competence is reflected in technical skills and general knowledge, pragmatic knowledge is knowledge about human activity, and reflective skills refer to the capacity to reflect critically on one's knowledge and experience. Although for Holiday and Chandler[6] wise persons will have general competence, will possess knowledge about human activity, and are able to reflect on their knowledge and experience, it is not clear how much of each of these components is necessary for a person to be wise.

In their conception of wisdom Baltes and his associates have largely ignored the role of reflection and have emphasised general competence and pragmatic knowledge.[7] Wisdom is defined as "an expert knowledge system in the fundamental pragmatics of life permitting exceptional insight, judgment, and advice involving complex and uncertain matters of the human condition."[8] These authors further note that "the body of knowledge and skills called wisdom involves a fine-tuned co-ordination of cognition, motivation, and emotion."

Underpinning the gaining of wisdom Baltes and his collaborators[9] argue a dual-process framework of intelligence. Two categories of intellect are distinguished by Baltes and his collaborators,[10] *fluid mechanics* and *crystallised mechanics*. *Fluid mechanics* encompasses the cognitive processes and structures underlying perception, memory, and classification. *Crystallised mechanics* comprise cultural knowledge and the application of knowledge derived from an individual's perceptual, memorial, and classification processes. This dual-process framework of intelligence is similar to, and has been influenced by, the crystallised and fluid intelligence of Cattell[11] and Horn.[12]

Fluid mechanics are susceptible to biological aging from early adulthood. Research has shown that from 10 years of age sensory activities are gradually declining but from 40 years onwards that decline accelerates rapidly.[13] Aging brings with it a decreased capacity to focus and sustain attention,[14] the ability to detect changes in the direction of motion and estimating distance and speed.[15] Older persons are less efficient in perceiving relations and classifications, slower in organising incoming information and less able to adopt different strategies to remember information.[16]

In contrast to *fluid mechanics, crystallised mechanics* may, at least through to late middle years, be enhanced with age. With increasing age the opportunities to acquire knowledge about the culture and apply that knowledge increases. This knowledge includes factual knowledge, knowledge about oneself, knowledge about other people, such as one's values and goals and those of other persons, knowledge about society such as its structure and its processes, and knowledge about strategies to optimise one's knowledge. It is this knowledge which is the basis of insight and which gives one the capacity to advise others on complex and uncertain matters including interpersonal relations.

One important implication of the dual-process model of intelligence is that whether one becomes wiser with age depends on age-related changes in both *fluid* and *crystallised mechanics*. Thus, during childhood and adolescence both the *fluid* and the *crystallised mechanics* will be positively correlated to the growth of knowledge and skills which underlie wisdom. However, in later life when cognitive processes and structures are impaired through biological aging, wisdom will not increase unless gains in cultural knowledge outweigh losses caused by the biological aging. Baltes[17] argues that the older an individual is, the more that individual is dependent on cultural artefacts to maintain high levels of functioning. Examples of present day cultural artefacts include such things as the internet, email, computers, medical technology, organisational hierarchies in business and government, and economic systems. This view of ontogenetic development is analogous to that proposed by Medawar[18] concerning phylogenetic development. Medawar maintained that the rapid development of the human species over the last several thousand years is a consequence of the development of techniques rather than genes. Survival of the species depends on the inheritance from the cultural pool and not the gene pool.

However, it would be erroneous to conclude that cultural factors always advantage older persons. In fact, cultural factors may act to the detriment of the very old. Western societies, driven by technological, scientific, and economic development, are changing with ever increasing rapidity. Not only does knowledge quickly become obsolete and skills become outmoded, many values and attitudes central to earlier eras become irrelevant. In Western societies significant changes have occurred and are occurring in social structure and social expectation, for example, the role of the family, the roles of women and men, permanence of employment, and the relevance of religion. Nor in today's society can one place too much reliance on cultural artefacts with which one has become familiar to compensate for the effects of biological aging because artefacts become obsolete. Culture is rapidly evolving. Therefore to enable effective use of culture, one must be able to acquire new knowledge, to learn new skills, and to adapt to new demands. However, the capacity to learn new skills is limited by biological aging. Neuronal plasticity decreases with age,[19] learning requires more time and effort and the level attained by old persons seldom matches that of the young.[20]

Thus, in industrialised western societies there is little scope for older persons to be the repository of relevant technical skills, since the technical skills and the knowledge of older persons are likely to have become obsolete. This state of affairs contrasts with that of non-industrial societies where much of the knowledge and skills within those societies are the same from one generation to the next and these skills and knowledge can be and are transmitted to the young by older generations.[21] It is in these societies that the knowledge of older persons is accepted as a valuable asset and it is from the ranks of the older persons that the members of the ruling council are generally drawn, the *elders* of the society.

For many, the hallmark of wise persons is not their possession of expertise in technical or interpersonal matters but their reflective skills.[22] One can acquire great competence or technical skills and become a technical expert, through experience one can acquire extensive knowledge about human activity and become an expert in knowing about human activities. But unless one can reflect on that expert knowledge, and see that knowledge in relation to broader issues, that is, one can see a "big picture," one has not become wise. Csikszentmihalyi and Rathunde[23] also make this point with the following example:

> It took marvellous ingenuity to invent aerosol sprays based on chlorofluorocarbons–the knowledge that went into this artifact puts all the philosophers in ancient Greece to shame. But how wise will this invention turn out to be if it destroys part of the ozone layer surrounding the planet, causing the harmful ultraviolet components of sunrays to kill much of the life inside the sea and to kill us through skin cancer? Measured against such effects, clean windows and odorless underarms does not seem such a bargain. If wisdom is a process by which people try to evaluate the ultimate consequences of events in terms of each other, it is more necessary now than Plato could have anticipated it to be over two millennia ago.

Both Kitchener and Brenner[24] and Arlin[25] have reached a similar conclusion about the central role that reflection plays in the acquiring of wisdom. Reflection allows one to reflect on experiences and to learn from one's mistakes. Through reflection one is able to know the limits of one's knowledge and the limits of human knowledge.

While there may be little difficulty in accepting that intelligence, technical skills, experience and reflection are all necessary ingredients to the acquisition of wisdom, there are still many issues left unresolved. How much intelligence, technical skills, and experience are necessary to become wise? What level of reflection is required? How big must the "big picture" be?

These questions raise other questions in their train. As with other human dispositions such as honesty, generosity, and kindness, is it a mistake to refer to someone as wise without contextualising that disposition. Thus, someone may be wise with respect to matters to do with human relationships but foolish in financial matters. A person whose decisions might be considered wise today might tomorrow be judged quite differently.

One inescapable conclusion to be drawn is that in an industrial society with rapid technological and social changes it is increasingly difficult to be wise across a broad range of areas, as it might previously have been. Equally, it is increasingly unlikely that individuals will be recognised as being wise across a community as a whole. Further, the currency of a person's actions as being judged wise is likely to be inversely related to the rate of technical and social change.

AGING AND WISDOM

What the relationship is between wisdom and aging depends very much on how wisdom is defined. If wisdom comprises two components: the capacity to quickly seize up a situation *and* then relate past experiences to that situation to provide solutions or insights to that situation, then whatever factors impact on those two components will be relevant to the gaining or losing of wisdom. Thus, a person who is slow to seize up a situation is unlikely to respond in a manner that is seen as wise. Similarly, a person who lacks experience is unlikely to be able to make a contribution that would be deemed wise.

In a western industrialised society very few people are likely to be recognised as wise. Thus, the young are unlikely to be wise or to be considered wise because they have acquired insufficient knowledge and experience and they have not developed skills to reflect. Potentially, people of middle years are well placed to act wisely as they have accrued knowledge and life experience and the impact of biological aging is not yet all pervasive. However, the day to day demands of living in an industrialised society are likely to limit the time and opportunity for reflection. Elderly persons may have the time and opportunity to reflect but their capacity to contribute to providing wise counsel is limited by the fact that their world is a different world from that of contemporary society. It is probably true to say that because social and interpersonal issues change less than technical ones, there is a greater probability that the elderly can contribute this wise counsel in the social and interpersonal domains. It will be those older persons whose intelligence, knowledge, and experience has not been outweighed by the effects of biological aging who will be in the best position to be wise. They can place present issues in a broader context than those who have a shorter life experience.

NOTES

1. Freeman, M.D.A., "Towards a critical theory of family law," *Current Legal Problems* (1985):153.

2. H.J. Chandler and S. Holiday, "Wisdom in a postapocalyptic age," in *Wisdom: Its Nature, Origin and Development,* edited by R.J. Sternberg (Cambridge, England: Cambridge University Press, 1990).

3. P.B. Baltes, "Theoretical propositions of life-span developmental psychology. On the dynamics of growth and decline," in *Developmental Psychology* 23 (1987): 611-626; P.B. Baltes, "On the incomplete architecture of human ontogeny: Selection, optimisation, and compensation as a foundation of developmental theory," *American Psychologist* 52 (1997): 366-380; P.B. Baltes, S.W. Cornelius, A. Spiro, J.R. Nesselroade and S.L. Willis, "Integration vs differentiation of fluid-crystallized intelligence in old age," *Developmental Psychology* 16 (1980): 625-635; P.B. Baltes and U. Lindenberger, "Emergence of a powerful connection between sensory and cognitive functioning across the adult life span: A new window at the study of cognitive aging," *Psychology and Aging* 12 (1997): 12-21; P.B. Baltes, J. Smith and U.M. Staudinger, "Wisdom and successful aging," in *The Nebraska Symposium on Motivation: The Psychology of Aging* 39, edited by H.T. Sonderegger (1992); P.B. Baltes and U.M. Staudinger, "The search for a psychology of wisdom," *Current Directions in Psychological Science* 2 (1993): 75-80; P.B. Baltes, U.M. Staudinger, A. Maercker and J. Smith, "People nominated as wise: A comparative study of wisdom-related knowledge," *Psychology and Aging* 10 (1995): 155-166; U. Lindenberger and P.B. Baltes, "Intellectual functioning in old and very old age: Cross-sectional results from the Berlin Aging Study," *Psychology and Aging* 12 (1997): 410-432; J. Smith and P.B. Baltes, "Wisdom-related knowledge: Age/cohort differences in response to life-planning problems," *Developmental Psychology* 26 (1990): 594-505; J. Smith and P.B. Baltes, "Profiles of psychological functioning in the old and the oldest old," *Psychology and Aging* 12 (1997): 458-472; U.M. Staudinger, J. Smith and P.B. Baltes, "Wisdom-related knowledge in a life review task: Age differences and the role of professional specialization," *Psychology and Aging* 7 (1992): 271-281.

4. P.K. Arlin, "Wisdom: The art of problem solving," in *Wisdom: Its Nature, Origin and Development*, edited by R.J. Sternberg (Cambridge, England: Cambridge University Press, 1990); Chandler and Holiday, "Wisdom in a postapocalyptic age"; V. Clayton, "Erickson's theory of human development as it applies to the aged: Wisdom as contradictive cognition," *Human Development* 18 (1975): 119-128; V. Clayton, "Wisdom and intelligence: The nature and function of knowledge in later years," *International Journal of Aging and Human Development* 15 (1982): 315-321; M. Csikszentmihalyi and K. Rathunde, "The psychology of wisdom: An evolutionary perspective," in *Wisdom: Its Nature, Origin, and Development*, edited by R.J. Sternberg (Cambridge, England: Cambridge University Press, 1990); S.G. Holiday and S.J. Chandler, *Wisdom: Explorations in adult competence* (Basel, Switzerland: Karger, 1986); K.S. Kitchener and H.G. Brenner, "Wisdom and reflective judgment: Knowing in the face of uncertainty," in *Wisdom: Its Nature, Origin, and Development*, edited by R.J. Sternberg (Cambridge, England: Cambridge University Press, 1990); G. Labouvie-Vief, "Wisdom as integrated thought: Historical and developmental perspectives," in *Wisdom: Its Nature, Origin, and Development*, edited by R.J. Sternberg (Cambridge, England: Cambridge University Press, 1990); J. Meacham, "The loss of wisdom," in *Wisdom: Its Nature, Origin, and Development*, edited by R.J. Sternberg (Cambridge, England: Cambridge University Press, 1990); R.J. Sternberg, "Implicit theories of intelligence, creativity, and wisdom," *Journal of Personality and Social Psychology* 49 (1985): 607-627.

5. Holiday and Chandler, *Wisdom: Explorations in adult competence.*

6. Ibid.

7. Baltes, "Theoretical propositions of life-span developmental psychology," 611-626; Baltes, "On the incomplete architecture of human ontogeny," 366-380; Baltes et al., "Integration vs differentiation," 625-635; Baltes and Lindenberger, "Emergence of a powerful connection," 12-21; Baltes et al., "Wisdom and successful aging"; Baltes and Staudinger, "The search for a psychology of wisdom," 75-80; Baltes et al., "People nominated as wise," 155-166; Lindenberger and Baltes, "Intellectual functioning in old and very old age," 410-432; Smith and Baltes, "Wisdom-related knowledge: Age/cohort differences," 594-505; Smith and Baltes, "Profiles of psychological functioning," 458-472; Staudinger et al., "Wisdom-related knowledge in a life review task," 271-281.

8. Baltes and Staudinger, "The search for a psychology of wisdom."

9. Baltes, "Theoretical propositions of life-span developmental psychology," 611-626; Baltes, "On the incomplete architecture of human ontogeny," 366-380; P.B. Baltes and J. Smith, "Toward a psychology of wisdom and its ontogenesis," in *Wisdom: Its Nature, Origins, and Development*, edited by R.J. Sternberg (Cambridge, England: Cambridge University Press, 1990); Baltes and Staudinger, "The search for a psychology of wisdom," 75-80; Smith and Baltes, "Wisdom-related knowledge: Age/cohort differences," 594-505.

10. Baltes, "Theoretical propositions of life-span developmental psychology," 611-626; Baltes, "On the incomplete architecture of human ontogeny," 366-380; Baltes and Staudinger, "The search for a psychology of wisdom," 75-80; Baltes et al., "Wisdom and successful aging."

11. R.B. Cattell, *Abilities: Their structure, growth and action* (Boston: Houghten Mifflin, 1971).

12. J.L. Horn, "Organisation of data a life span development of human abilities," in *Lifespan development psychology: Research and theory,* edited by L.R. Goulet and P.B. Beles (New: Academic Press, 1970), 423-466.

13. A.J. Adams, L.S. Wong, L. Wong and B. Gould, "Visual acuity changes with age," *American Journal of Optometry and Physiological Optics* 65 (1988): 403; H. Davis and S.R. Silverman, *Hearing and Deafness* (Holt, Reinhart and Winston, 1960); C.J. Owsley, R. Sekuler and D. Siemsen, "Contrast sensitivity throughout adulthood," *Vision Research* 23 (1983): 689; R. Sekuler and R. Blake, *Perception* (McGraw-Hill, 1990).

14. L.M. Giambra and R.E. Quilter, "Sustained attention in adulthood: A unique, large sample, large sample longitudinal multicohort analysis using the Mackworth Clock test," *Psychology and Aging* 3 (1988): 75; D.J. Madden, "Adult differences in attentional capacity demands of visual search," *Cognitive Development* 1 (1986): 335; D.J. Madden, "Aging, attention, and the use of hearing during visual search," *Cognitive Development* 2 (1987): 201; R.E. Quilter, L.H. Giambra, and P.E. Benson, "Longitudinal age changes in vigilance over an eighteen year interval," *Journal of Gerontology* 38 (1983): 51.

15. K. Ball and R. Sekuler, "Improving visual perception in observers," *Journal of Gerontology* 41 (1986): 176; C.T. Scialfa,. L.T. Guzy, H.W. Leibowitz, P.M. Garvey and R.A. Tyrell, "Age differences in estimating vehicle velocity," *Psychology and Aging* 6 (1991): 60.

16. F.I.M. Craik, "Age differences in human memory," in *Handbook of the Psychology of Aging,* edited by J.E. Birren and K.W. Schiae (Van Nostrand Reinhold, 1977); F.I.M. Craik and J.C. Rabinowitz, "Age differences in the acquisition and use of verbal information," in *Attention and Performance* 10, edited by J.Long and A. Baddley (Erlbaum, 1984); D.H. Kausler, *Experimental Psychology and Human Aging* (Wiley, 1982); D.M. Thomson and R. Gannon, "The encoding specificity paradigm: A diagnostic test," in *Brain Impairment,* Proceedings of the 1984 Annual Brain Impairment Conference, Melbourne, Australian Society for the Study of Brain Impairment, edited by M. Field, J. Hendy, C. Roberts and P. Hopkins (1985).

17. Baltes, "On the incomplete architecture of human ontogeny," 366-380.

18. P.C. Medawar, "Onwards from Spencer: Evolution and evolutionism," *Encounter* 21 (1963): 35-43.

19. D. Magnusson, ed., *The lifespan development of individuals: Behavioural, neurobiological, and psychosocial perspectives* (Cambridge, England: Cambridge University Press, 1996).

20. P.B. Baltes and R. Kliegel, "Further testing of limits of cognitive plasticity: Negative age differences in a mnemonic skill are robust," *Developmental Psychology* 28 (1992): 121-125; Baltes and Lindenberger, "Emergence of a powerful connection between sensory and cognitive functioning," 12-21; P. Rendell and D.M. Thomson, "Aging and prospective memory: Differences between naturalistic and laboratory tastes," *Journal of Gerontology: Psychological Sciences* 54b (1999): 256-269; D.M. Thomson and R. Gannon, "The encoding specificity paradigm: A diagnostic test," in *Brain Impairment,* Proceedings of the 1984 Annual Brain Impairment Conference, Melbourne, Australian Society for the Study of Brain Impairment, edited by M. Field, J. Hendy, C. Roberts and P. Hopkins (1985).

21. J.S. Bruner, *Studies in Cognitive Growth* (New York: Wiley, 1966).

22. Arlin, "Wisdom: The art of problem solving"; Chandler and Holiday, "Wisdom in a postapocalyptic age"; V. Clayton, "Wisdom and intelligence: The nature and func-

tion of knowledge in later years," *International Journal of Aging and Human Development* 15 (1982): 315-321; V.P. Clayton and J.E. Birren, "The development of wisdom across the lifespan: A re-examination of an ancient topic," in *Lifespan development and behavior* 3, edited by P.B. Baltes and O.G. Brim (New York: Academic Press, 1980),103-135; Csikszentmihalyi and Rathunde, "The psychology of wisdom: an evolutionary perspective"; Chandler and Holiday, "Wisdom in a post apocalyptic age"; Kitchener and Brenner, "Wisdom and reflective judgment."

23. Csikszentmihalyi and Rathunde, "The psychology of wisdom: An evolutionary perspective."

24. Kitchener and Brenner, "Wisdom and reflective judgment."

25. Arlin, "Wisdom: The art of problem solving."

REFERENCES

Adams, A.J., L.S Wong, L. Wong, and B. Gould, "Visual acuity changes with age." *American Journal of Optometry and Physiological Optics* 65 (1988): 403.

Arlin, P.K. "Wisdom: The art of problem solving." In *Wisdom: Its Nature, Origin, and Development*, edited by R.J. Sternberg. Cambridge, England: Cambridge University Press, 1990.

Ball, K., and R. Sekuler, "Improving visual perception in observers." *Journal of Gerontology* 41 (1986): 176.

Baltes, P.B. "Theoretical propositions of life-span developmental psychology. On the dynamics of growth and decline." *Developmental Psychology* 23 (1987): 611-626.

Baltes, P.B. "On the incomplete architecture of human ontogeny: Selection, optimisation, and compensation as a foundation of developmental theory." *American Psychologist* 52 (1997): 366-380.

Baltes, P.B., S.W. Cornelius, A. Spiro, J.R. Nesselroade, and S.L. Willis. "Integration vs differentiation of fluid-crystallized intelligence in old age." *Developmental Psychology* 16 (1980): 625-635.

Baltes, P.B., and U. Lindenberger. "Emergence of a powerful connection between sensory and cognitive functioning across the adult life span: A new window at the study of cognitive aging." *Psychology and Aging* 12 (1997): 12-21.

Baltes, P.B., and R. Kliegel. "Further testing of limits of cognitive plasticity: Negative age differences in a mnemonic skill are robust." *Developmental Psychology* 28 (1992): 121-125.

Baltes, P.B., and J. Smith. "Toward a psychology of wisdom and its ontogenesis." In *Wisdom: Its Nature, Origins, and Development*, edited by R.J. Sternberg. Cambridge, England: Cambridge University Press, 1990.

Baltes, P.B., and J. Smith. "A systemic-wholistic view of psychological functioning in very old: Introduction to a collection of articles from the Berlin Aging Study." *Psychology and Aging* 12 (1997): 395-409.

Baltes, P.B., and U.M. Staudinger. "The search for a psychology of wisdom." *Current Directions in Psychological Science* 2 (1993): 75-80.

Baltes, P.B., J. Smith, and U.M. Staudinger. "Wisdom and successful aging." In *The Nebraska Symposium on Motivation: The Psychology of Aging*, vol. 39, edited by H.T. Sonderegger (1992).

Baltes, P.B., U.M. Staudinger, A. Maercker, and J. Smith. "People nominated as wise: A comparative study of wisdom-related knowledge." *Psychology and Aging* 10 (1995): 155-166.

Bruner, J.S. *Studies in Cognitive Growth*. New York: Wiley, 1966.

Cattell, R.B. *Abilities: Their structure, growth and action*. Boston: Houghten Mifflin, 1971.

Chandler, H.J., and S. Holiday. "Wisdom in a postapocalyptic age." In *Wisdom: Its Nature, Origins and Development*, edited by R.J. Sternberg. Cambridge, England: Cambridge University Press, 1990.

Clayton, V. "Erickson's theory of human development as it applies to the aged: Wisdom as contradictive cognition." *Human Development* 18 (1975): 119-128.

Clayton, V. "Wisdom and intelligence: The nature and function of knowledge in later years." *International Journal of Aging and Human Development* 15 (1982): 315-321.

Clayton, V.P., and J.E Birren. "The development of wisdom across the lifespan: A re-examination of an ancient topic." In *Lifespan development and behaviour*, vol. 3, edited by P.B. Baltes and O.G. Brim, 103-135. New York: Academic Press, 1980.

Craik, F.I.M. "Age differences in human memory." In *Handbook of the Psychology of Aging*, edited by J.E. Birren and K.W. Schiae. Van Nostrand Reinhold, 1977.

Craik, F.I.M., and J.C. Rabinowitz. "Age differences in the acquisition and use of verbal information." In *Attention and Performance*, vol. 10, edited by J. Long and A. Baddley. Erlbaum, 1984.

Csikszentmihalyi, M., and K Rathunde. "The psychology of wisdom: An evolutionary perspective." In *Wisdom: Its Nature, Origin, and Development*, edited by R.J. Sternberg. Cambridge, England: Cambridge University Press, 1990.

Davis, H., and S.R. Silverman. *Hearing and Deafness*. Holt, Reinhart and Winston, 1960.

Freeman, M.D.A. "Towards a critical theory of family law," *Current Legal Problems* (1985): 153.

Giambra, L.M., and R.E. Quilter. "Sustained attention in adulthood: A unique, large sample, large sample longitudinal multicohort analysis using the Mackworth Clock test." *Psychology and Aging* 3 (1988): 75.

Heckhausen, J., R. Dixon, and P.B. Baltes. "Gains and losses in development throughout adulthood as perceived by different adult age groups." *Development Psychology* 25 (1989): 109-121.

Holiday, S.G., and S.J. Chandler. *Wisdom: Explorations in adult competence*. Basel, Switzerland: Karger, 1986.

Horn, J.L. "Organisation of data a life span development of human abilities." In *Life-span development psychology: Research and theory*, edited by L.R. Goulet and P.B. Beles. New: Academic Press, 1970, 423-466.

Kausler, D.H. *Experimental Psychology and Human Aging*. Wiley, 1982.

Kitchener, K.S., and H.G. Brenner. "Wisdom and reflective judgment: Knowing in the face of uncertainty." In *Wisdom: Its Nature, Origin, and Development*, edited by R.J. Sternberg. Cambridge, England: Cambridge University Press, 1990.

Labouvie-Vief, G. "Wisdom as integrated thought: Historical and developmental perspectives." In *Wisdom: Its Nature, Origin, and Development*, edited by R.J. Sternberg. Cambridge, England: Cambridge University Press, 1990.

Lindenberger, U., and P.B. Baltes. "Intellectual functioning in old and very old age: Cross-sectional results from the Berlin Aging Study." *Psychology and Aging* 12 (1997): 410-432.

Madden, D.J. "Adult differences in attentional capacity demands of visual search." *Cognitive Development* 1 (1986): 335.

Madden, D.J. "Aging, attention, and the use of hearing during visual search." *Cognitive Development* 2 (1987): 201.

Magnusson D., ed. *The lifespan development of individuals: Behavioral, neurobiological, and psychosocial perspectives.* Cambridge, England: Cambridge University Press, 1996.

Meacham, J. "The loss of wisdom." In *Wisdom: Its Nature, Origin, and Development*, edited by R.J. Sternberg. Cambridge, England: Cambridge University Press, 1990.

Medawar, P.C. "Onwards from Spencer: Evolution and evolutionism." *Encounter* 21 (1963): 35-43.

Owsley, C.J., R. Sekuler, and D. Siemsen. "Contrast sensitivity throughout adulthood," *Vision Research* 23 (1983): 689.

Quilter, R.E., L.H. Giambra, and P.E. Benson. "Longitudinal age changes in vigilance over an eighteen year interval." *Journal of Gerontology* 38 (1983): 51.

Rendell, P., and D.M. Thomson. "Aging and prospective memory: Differences between naturalistic and laboratory tastes." *Journal of Gerontology: Psychological Sciences* 54b (1999): 256-269.

Scialfa, C.T., L.T. Guzy, H.W. Leibowitz, P.M. Garvey, and R.A. Tyrell. "Age differences in estimating vehicle velocity." *Psychology and Aging* 6 (1991): 60.

Sekuler, R., and R. Blake *Perception*. McGraw-Hill, 1990.

Smith, J., and P.B. Baltes. "Wisdom-related knowledge: Age/cohort differences in response to life-planning problems." *Developmental Psychology* 26 (1990): 594-505.

Smith, J. and P.B. Baltes. "Profiles of psychological functioning in the old and the oldest old." *Psychology and Aging* 12 (1997): 458-472.

Staudinger, U. M., J. Smith, and P.B. Baltes. "Wisdom-related knowledge in a life review task: Age differences and the role of professional specialization." *Psychology and Aging* 7 (1992): 271-281.

Sternberg, R.J. "Implicit theories of intelligence, creativity, and wisdom." *Journal of Personality and Social Psychology* 49 (1985): 607-627.

Thomson D.M., and R. Gannon. "The encoding specificity paradigm: A diagnostic test." In *Brain Impairment*, Proceedings of the 1984 Annual Brain Impairment Conference, Melbourne, Australian Society for the Study of Brain Impairment, edited by M. Field, J. Hendy, C. Roberts, and P. Hopkins (1985).

SECTION 2:
ISSUES OF AGEING
AND PASTORAL CARE

Ageing and Isolation:
Is the Issue Social Isolation
or Is It Lack of Meaning in Life?

Elizabeth MacKinlay, RN, PhD

SUMMARY. Social and spiritual isolation are growing issues for an ageing society that promotes the ideals of autonomy and high levels of individuation amongst its citizens. This chapter explores the issues of social and spiritual isolation for older adults and ways of addressing these issues both now and in the future. The need for intimacy with God and with others is illustrated using material from in-depth interviews with older

Rev. Dr. Elizabeth MacKinlay is Senior Lecturer at University of Canberra, Australia, Director of the Centre for Ageing and Pastoral Studies, at St. Mark's National Theological Centre, Canberra, and honorary assistant priest at the Anglican Church of the Good Shepherd, ACT.

The second study was supported by the Anglican Diocesan Foundation, Diocese of Canberra and Goulburn and Anglican Retirement Community Services (ARCS) Canberra and Goulburn.

Material in this chapter is based on material published in "The Spiritual Dimension of Ageing" (2000) Jessica Kingsley Publishers. Permission granted to print.

[Haworth co-indexing entry note]: "Ageing and Isolation: Is the Issue Social Isolation or Is It Lack of Meaning in Life?" MacKinlay, Elizabeth. Co-published simultaneously in *Journal of Religious Gerontology* (The Haworth Pastoral Press, an imprint of The Haworth Press, Inc.) Vol. 12, No. 3/4, 2001, pp. 89-99; and: *Aging, Spirituality and Pastoral Care: A Multi-National Perspective* (ed: Elizabeth MacKinlay, James W. Ellor, and Stephen Pickard) The Haworth Pastoral Press, an imprint of The Haworth Press, Inc., 2001, pp. 89-99. Single or multiple copies of this article are available for a fee from The Haworth Document Delivery Service [1-800-342-9678, 9:00 a.m. - 5:00 p.m. (EST). E-mail address: getinfo@haworthpressinc.com].

adults who live independently and others who are residents of aged care facilities. *[Article copies available for a fee from The Haworth Document Delivery Service: 1-800-342-9678. E-mail address: <getinfo@haworthpressinc.com> Website: <http://www.HaworthPress.com> © 2001 by The Haworth Press, Inc. All rights reserved.]*

KEYWORDS. Ageing, social isolation, spiritual isolation, intimacy, failure to thrive, spiritual resources

AGEING, SOCIAL ISOLATION AND LONELINESS

Australian Bureau of Statistics (ABS) projections state one in six people in Canberra will be living alone by 2021.[1] This includes all age groups; however, the majority of these will be older adults. Is living alone an issue for older people and what proportion of these people are socially isolated? An important question may be asked: Is the major issue social isolation, or is it a lack of meaning in life? It is appropriate to ask these questions at a time when society is ageing and more and more older people are living alone.

In both North American and Australian societies the importance of individuation is stressed, but, according to Bellah, "Absolute independence is a false ideal. It delivers not the autonomy it promises but loneliness and vulnerability instead."[2] At least some older adults may find the concept of independence increasingly difficult to maintain.

Rubinstein, Kilbride and Nagy found in a study of frail older adults living alone in the USA, that even though they all experienced severe health problems, generally had low incomes, were socially marginalised and had few social supports, 86% reported they lived alone by choice.[3] A major study conducted for the Commonwealth Department of Veterans' Affairs by Gardner, Brooke, Ozanne and Kendig, identified social isolation as an issue for the whole of the Australian community.[4] In their research they found that within the veteran community there was an overall problem of social isolation of approximately 10% isolated with another 12% at risk of isolation.

In studies of older people living independently or as residents in nursing homes I found that *some* of those living alone were socially isolated, while others were not.[5] In-depth interviews were used to gain insight into the ways in which these people were able to find meaning in life and to map their spirituality in later life. Spirituality as I write about it here recognises the sphere of ultimate meaning in people's lives, the meaning which arises from the core of one's being. Meaning for these older adults has often been found in relationship.

So, what is the relationship, if any, between loneliness, social isolation and spiritual isolation? It was found in one study that is possible for spiritual and social isolation to be present together, but also possible to be socially isolated without being spiritually isolated.[6]

This raises the questions of the need for human relationship and relationship with God, and asks why is it that some feel spiritually satisfied even while experiencing social isolation, and indeed why some are both socially and spiritually isolated, and have no sense of life satisfaction. The process of sanctification as described by Tillich can be used to gain some understanding of this.[7] The third principle that Tillich refers to is increasing relatedness and is relevant to the discussion of social and spiritual isolation:

> Only a relation which is inherent in all other relations, and which can even exist without them, is able to do so. Sanctification, or the process toward Spiritual maturity, conquers loneliness by providing for solitude and communion in interdependence. A decisive symptom of Spiritual maturity is the power to sustain solitude. Sanctification conquers introversion by turning the personal centre . . . toward the dimension of its depth and its height. Relatedness needs the vertical dimension in order to actualise itself in the horizontal dimension.[8]

What Tillich has described here is seen in the stories of some of the informants that follow. Carol says she has few friends and is socially isolated, but has developed a deep sense of spirituality and relationship with God and is not spiritually isolated. Carol has a real sense of meaning in her life based on her spiritual maturity. George and Win also fit this description, although Win also enjoys some social interaction. Helga, on the other hand, has neither social nor spiritual satisfaction. She feels lonely and isolated and she continues to search for both human relationship and some sense of "other" that she can relate to.

It was found in these studies that where the individual had a deep sense of spirituality and a well developed set or portfolio of spiritual strategies, social isolation did not seem to have the same impact.[9] Effective spiritual portfolios included deep and personal relationship with God, prayer, worship, study of a spiritual nature, and for some reading of Scripture and regular meditation.

Intimacy in Later Life

Meaning expressed through human relationship involves support and the need for connection with others. That quality of relationship can best be described as the need for intimacy, important at any time during the life cycle, and no less so in ageing.

Carroll and Dyckman describe intimacy as "the ability to let myself be known by another and to be comfortable in that revelation . . . At the deepest core of my being I need to be known and loved as I am."[10] Intimacy is touching deeply into another human being, connecting at a deep level. They see this as a safe place to be, without the need for masks and inhibitions, and acknowledge this as a reciprocal need. The need for intimacy was clearly expressed by some of the informants in my studies. The human need for intimacy is at its deepest an expression of the spiritual dimension.

For any single older adults, whether never married, widowed, separated or divorced, the need for confidantes and intimates arises. Indeed, living alone and housebound may be a form of involuntary solitary isolation. Yet moving to a hostel or nursing home does not necessarily solve the problems of loneliness. Katie, a resident in a nursing home, spoke of feeling really down at times, how she needed to talk to someone about her life and its meaning, and to work things through: "There's nobody . . . I've just got to think things out for myself. . . . it's a lonely life for one person to come into a big place like this." She went on:

> I'm on a lonely scale as a matter of fact, because my daughter had to have an operation for her heart and I can't see her and I don't ever see her daughter, she's only got the one, and I've got nobody in Canberra that I know. They just gave me 24 hours notice to come here and they have done a lot for me since I've been here, I'm much better.[11]

Katie said that she often wishes there was someone she could talk to about her life:

> No, it makes it very hard, you know. . . . There are often times you feel like a talk even if you go back over the years, just something different, because I can't see well enough to read now and I've just got to live this . . . no one to talk to or no one that I know, I've just got to lay there and think things out and try and work out something but it's almost impossible when you can't . . . you don't know anybody.

Katie's sense of isolation was clear, it seemed too that she was at-tempting to search for final meanings in her life; she was reminiscing, and wanted someone to help her and perhaps journey with her in this task. As she rightly said, there was no one in the nursing home who could do that with her. Time constraints and staffing would not allow for this. Her prayer life was well developed and she regularly prayed, thanking God:

> I do thank God for all He has done for me in the time that I've been with Him. Sometimes it seems hard that you should be left on your own then I think well, there's a reason for it, because I think He has a reason for us all. I do really! It mightn't suit us always.

Here Katie expressed both grief over the loss of her marriage and her thankfulness for her relationship with God. Katie's need for relation-ship with others was partly fulfilled by her attending every church ser-vice that was held in the nursing home, of any denomination. However, it is noted this did not fulfil her needs for an intimate relationship with another human being.

The loss of intimate relationships in later life is common. Being alone in later life is even more common for women than men. It is rather obvi-ous that experience of widowhood becomes more likely with increasing age. Doris, a widow said, "the grief . . . when one loses one's husband, is something that rocks your life to its very foundations": Her husband died nine years ago. Doris now has a deep self-understanding and re-cognises her need for someone to share with on a spiritual base; and she acknowledges she has such a relationship. Although the death of her husband was a major loss in her life, she has rebuilt her life and relation-ships. One of the ways Doris has rebuilt relationships is through in-volvement in a long term Christian group; they have been meeting regularly for eight years. This is a great source of comfort and a place where she can also continue to grow spiritually.[12]

Living Alone and the Possibility of Social Isolation

Social isolation was not found to be dependent on living alone. Some participants in the study had lived alone all their adult lives. The ways they were managing at the time of interview varied a great deal.

One never married frail woman (Carol) living alone said that ade-quate social support was becoming a real issue.[13] She said she couldn't rely on human contacts, "People die and children move away." I asked her how she felt about this. She replied, "It's scary." Then she went on to say, "But it throws you back on yourself, and a need to explore your own depth." This was a continuing spiritual journey for her. She had developed a deep sense of meaning in her life. It seemed that for this woman being socially isolated was matched by further spiritual growth. Carol is certainly not spiritually isolated. However, Carol has been actively developing her spiritual life over a number of years. The strategies she uses provide her with a rich spiritual resource that go some way towards overcoming her social isolation. Among the strategies she uses on a regular basis are prayer, reading and study of religious books, and Christian meditation. She attends church but is dependent on having someone drive her to church.

George has never married, and says he never has regrets for choosing not to. He is definitely not socially isolated; in fact he draws a real distinction between being lonely and being alone. He appears to have sufficient resources within himself; perhaps one could say he has achieved a high level of individuation. He has contact with some friends and members of religious orders and his contemplation of their life style may be a factor here, it is difficult to say. His obvious interest in reading and writing are important factors in his life satisfaction and finding meaning.

Win, another never married, accepts that it is God's purpose in her life that she would never marry. Once having decided that, she accepted her decision and appears comfortable with it. Her emotional and spiritual supports are from sharing deeply with a woman whose husband is a resident in a nursing home. She recognises that her understanding of the spiritual has moved to a different level, a level at which she cannot share with some of the others. Christian meditation is a regular part of her week.

She told an anecdote of visiting a former resident of her village, who was now quite frail and in a nursing home. This story illustrated some of the depth of this woman's spirituality, her understanding, and acceptance of life, ability for relationship, and compassion:

> I'd had the thought to go over and see her that afternoon. . . . And so we had a wonderful talk about death and dying and she said, "I don't think I'll see my 95th birthday" or something like that, and I could tell she was, (Win paused). She said her legs were aching, so I said: "Well shall I rub your legs?" So I rubbed her legs, and the next day I heard that she'd died, and I thought I felt, well you

know, sad that she had died but I felt so grateful that I'd had that time with her before she died.

The time the two friends shared was obviously an important time of deep and open communication, and a seeming mutual recognition of the approaching death of Win's friend. There is a sense of the specialness of that last physical act she rendered to her friend, of rubbing her legs. Then the next day, when she heard of her friend's death, there was acceptance of the end of a life, and sadness. But there was also a sense of the grace present in the situation of the previous day; she was grateful that she had spent time with her friend so soon before she died.

Some Are More Equal Than Others When Living Alone

Two of those interviewed who had never married seemed to see themselves as different from the widowed group. It is possible that these two were unable to accept their situation and carried a sense of failure, based on societal expectations, probably more strongly held in that cohort of women, that women should marry. Isolation within church communities of those who are single was another factor to be negotiated for these never married women.

Although Dawn said that church had lost its meaning for her, she still attended. It might well be asked why she did, and it would seem one reason might be her sense of isolation. For Dawn and others like her the church community is perhaps more truly their family than for other members of the church. If they felt rejection here, then there seemed to be no other place to go.

Divorced and Socially Isolated

Helga's marriage broke down, a number of years ago. She says, she is very lonely, "Sex is good and healthy." She misses intimacy and the financial support of a relationship, and expressed the desire to be cared for. She says she has social support from a number of friends, but none really close at present. She then confided: "I still get hopelessly lonely, when I come into an empty flat in the evenings, and in the morning, because I haven't got many really close friends, just round here."

In fact, Helga seemed to have few inner resources to assist her overcome the loneliness that seemed to characterise her life. Her recent years have been marked by a continuing search for meaning in life, and a lack of satisfaction in this search.

FAILURE TO THRIVE AND AGEING

As we examine new ways of being society in an ageing society, it will be necessary to consider how friendships may be fostered for those who are older and live alone. The need for human intimacy is, it seems, also related to failure to thrive for at least some frail older people. The failure to thrive syndrome that has come onto the agenda through the gerontological literature in recent years, is of course borrowed from the paediatric literature. This syndrome describes a set of signs in some older people, including: loss of appetite, physical and cognitive disability and social and environmental impairment.[15] It is a condition that is seen in frail older people, in those with malnutrition, with dementia and delirium. I believe we must also bear in mind that there does come a time where physiological changes in the process of dying make it impossible to alter that dying trajectory. Thus it may be futile to try to reverse the physical decline.

Now I wonder how much of this may be related to lack of nourishment for the soul. If we are to consider holistic care, then this is a major challenge. Gerontological literature recognises it, do we take account of this in pastoral care and chaplaincy, and does parish nursing recognise it? Simply recognising and naming the syndrome is empowering. Once we have done that we have somewhere to go.

But I still have a concern that the spiritual needs may not be addressed unless those who make the diagnosis have that on their agenda. Perhaps this failure to thrive syndrome is really a loss of meaning in life.

In conducting in-depth interviews with frail older residents of nursing homes, I have found that often when first meeting an older resident, it may seem that there is little that the person may want to talk about. Observing some older people, it seems that they do not converse much at all. Of course many nursing home residents find communication complex due to sight and hearing deficits. But given an opportunity to talk, of having someone who can sit with them and listen, makes all the difference. Often nurses involved in studies of spirituality in nursing homes reported this.[16] They found when they interviewed people they cared for on a daily basis, asking them the deeper questions of meaning and concern was like "opening the flood gates."

The need of residents of nursing homes to have someone to share with them is very apparent. Good physical care and activity programs are important, but not enough. There is a need for holistic care, that involves forming trusting, intimate and respectful relationships. There is a need for effective pastoral care programs in residential aged care. These programs should include opportunities for older people to participate in spiritual reminiscence and deal with issues of guilt, regrets, need for forgiveness and reconciliation.

Having adequate spiritual resources or spiritual portfolios may be protective against isolation. In our current society I suspect that many people have not had nor taken opportunities to develop these over their life span. One challenge is to assist these people to develop the strategies they need to live effectively in the latter part of their lives. Part of this challenge is to examine the work of people such as Tillich to see how the process of sanctification may be developed or facilitated in older people. It would seem that people like Carol, whose story was discussed earlier in the chapter, have, through the disappointments and losses in human relationships, turned to God, perhaps even out of a sense of hopelessness, to find hope and meaning. That is the paradox of life, so clearly expressed by Jesus, when he said: "For those who want to save their life will lose it, and those who lose their life for my sake, and for the sake of the gospel, will save it."[17]

So, Is the Real Issue Social Isolation or Is It Lack of Meaning of Life?

With the current trends in society to encourage and facilitate living at home for more older people, and with the increase in numbers of older people in the population, the issues of both social and spiritual isolation will become more important. The issues may need to be addressed at multiple levels, of appropriate housing for older people, better community based services and just as importantly, dealing with the issue of spiritual isolation and meaning in life. If we fail these older people, and particularly the 'shut-ins,' they may be both socially and spiritually isolated in their own homes.

Some programs are now being used that reduce this fragmentation of services and provide more quality time for these people. I am thinking mainly of the Community Care Packages, that provide a range of services to enable older people to remain living in their own homes.[14] However, we are still addressing only part of the problem. In our technological era we have neglected to develop the spiritual dimension, so unless people have these strategies to find meaning in life in their 'shut-in' existence, then they may still face tremendous loneliness and isolation.

Older people who live alone may find opportunities for developing new intimacies in later life, relationships that may bring a new sense of meaning into their lives. But, in reality, in the current society, often there are not the opportunities for doing so. There are barriers to older people forming new sexual relationships and existing friendships in later life may be hard to maintain in a mobile society, let alone establishing new friendships. Jim Seeber takes up the theme of sexuality and ageing in the next chapter.

CONCLUSION

It was noted in these studies that there did not seem to be a direct link between living alone and being socially or indeed spiritually isolated. As well, it was possible to be lonely while being a resident of a nursing home, surrounded as it were, with people, both other residents and staff. Rather, it seemed that having a real sense of meaning in life was primary. That then influenced the person's attitudes to life. This sense of meaning for most informants grew out of relationship.

Relationship with God, and relationship with others, are both important dimensions of being human. For many, there seems to be a continuing move of self-transcendence and self-forgetting as part of the ageing process, where the need for relationship and connectedness with others becomes even more urgent. This move seems to correspond with that described by Tillich in sanctification, the move for increasing relatedness.

In a society where more and more people will be living alone, it is asked where will that relationship come from? New and creative ways of finding relationship with others will need to be fostered. For many older people living alone, the main way this occurs at present is through aged care services delivered to the home. However, bringing aged care services to the home does not necessarily meet these needs for relationship, where relationship means connecting deeply with others, that is meeting at the level of the spiritual.

But what of the possibilities of relationship with God? For some older people the deepening of spiritual relationship with God transcends the losses of other relationships, and brings the deepest of intimacies known to human beings. How often for frail older people is this a reality, how often does this occur and we as carers are not even aware of it? How often do older people long for connectedness with God, and fail to find it? How may this need for connectedness in frail older people be facilitated? There are many questions yet to be answered.

NOTES

1. Australian Bureau of Statistics, 2000 www.

2. R. Bellah, R. Madsen, W.M. Sullivan, A. Swidler, S.M. Tipton, *Habits of the Heart: Individualism and Commitment to American Life* (Berkeley: University of California Press, 1985).

3. R.L. Rubinstein, J.C. Kilbride, S. Nagy, *Elders Living Alone: Frailty and the Perception of Choice* (New York: Aldine De Gruyter, 1992).

4. I. Gardner, E. Brooke, E. Ozanne and H. Kendig, *Improving Social Networks: A Research Report* prepared for Commonwealth Department of Veterans' Affairs, 1999.

5. E.B. MacKinlay, "The Spiritual Dimension of Ageing: Meaning in Life, Response to Meaning and Well Being in Ageing" (doctoral thesis LaTrobe University, 1998).

6. Ibid.

7. P. Tillich, *Systematic Theology,* vol. 3 (Chicago: The University of Chicago Press, 1963).

8. Ibid., 234.

9. MacKinlay, "The Spiritual Dimension of Ageing."

10. L.P. Carroll, K.M. Dyckman, *Chaos or Creation: Spirituality in Mid-life* (New York: Paulist Press, 1986), 123.

11. E.B. MacKinlay, in-depth interviews completed 2000, of older adults resident in nursing homes in Canberra.

12. MacKinlay, "The Spiritual Dimension of Ageing."

13. Ibid.

14. Community Aged Care Packages, an initiative of the Federal Department of Aged Care, Canberra.

15. D.D. Groom, "A Diagnostic Model for Failure to Thrive," in *Journal of Gerontological Nursing* 19 (6), (1993): 12-16.

16. E.B. MacKinlay, "Spirituality and Ageing: Bringing Meaning to Life" in *St Mark's Review* (Canberra), no. 155 (Spring 1993): p. 26-30.

17. Mark 8:35.

Pastoral Support for Late-Life Sexuality

James J. Seeber, PhD, DMin

SUMMARY. As more persons live longer and enjoy relatively good physical health, new ethical questions arise. One set of questions regards the continuation of sexual life among older persons, especially among older unmarried persons. Women live many years longer than their spouses and often were of a younger age than the spouses. The Judeo-Christian tradition affirms the vitality of sex as a basic part of God's gift of physical creation. A large majority of older people view sexual expression as important and many see it as crucial to a good relationship with a partner. These issues are raised for the awareness of pastoral counselors to understand and be responsive to the varied sexual alternatives in the later years in order to offer practical help to older persons. *[Article copies available for a fee from The Haworth Document Delivery Service: 1-800-342-9678. E-mail address: <getinfo@ haworthpressinc.com> Website: <http://www.HaworthPress.com> © 2001 by The Haworth Press, Inc. All rights reserved.]*

KEYWORDS. Sexuality and aging, religion and sexuality, pastoral care and sexuality

---

James J. Seeber is Associate Director, Center for Aging, Religion and Spirituality, Luther Seminary, St. Paul, MN.

Address correspondence to: James J. Seeber, 409 East Graham Street, Bloomington, IL 61701 (E-mail: Jamesstuba@aol.com).

Appreciation is expressed to the Center for Aging in Pastoral Studies, St. Mark's Theological Centre, Canberra, ACT, Australia for the opportunity to present the original draft of this paper at the First International Conference on Pastoral Care and Aging in Canberra in January, 2000.

[Haworth co-indexing entry note]: "Pastoral Support for Late-Life Sexuality" Seeber, James J. Co-published simultaneously in *Journal of Religious Gerontology* (The Haworth Pastoral Press, an imprint of The Haworth Press, Inc.) Vol. 12, No. 3/4, 2001, pp. 101-109; and: *Aging, Spirituality and Pastoral Care: A Multi-National Perspective* (ed: Elizabeth MacKinlay, James W. Ellor, and Stephen Pickard) The Haworth Pastoral Press, an imprint of The Haworth Press, Inc., 2001, pp. 101-109. Single or multiple copies of this article are available for a fee from The Haworth Document Delivery Service [1-800-342-9678, 9:00 a.m. - 5:00 p.m. (EST). E-mail address: getinfo@haworthpressinc.com].

HARRY

It was in the busier days of winter that chaplain Joe noticed Harry had not been attending the weekly vespers service for some weeks. Harry, a quiet and thoughtful retired civil servant had come to vespers each Wednesday night when he and his wife had moved to the home. As her health declined, Harry became the chief caregiver until the dementia with which she suffered became more than Harry could manage alone. Upon the recommendation of staff members after a review of the situation, Harry's wife Betty was transferred to the nursing care center on campus where she seemed to adjust fairly well. Chaplain Joe noticed that Betty didn't remember who he was when he stopped in to say hello and her conversation, while reasonable, didn't square with reality. Betty spoke at times of getting back to the house to "fix dinner" but accepted residential life in the nursing home with out significant protests.

It worked well for Harry. He could stop by to see her a couple of times each day as the facility was only about 30 yards from the main campus dining room. After two or three months, however, rumors began to circulate that Harry had a girlfriend. He had been seen at one of the fine restaurants in the village having dinner with a woman, and later word had gone around that the girlfriend lived across the boulevard from Friendly Hills in the public housing units for older people. It was about then that Chaplain Joe noticed Harry's absence from vespers.

Discreetly discussing the matter with two of the professional staff members in the home, Chaplain Joe wondered if he should contact Harry. The nurse reported that Harry was not ill. He was stopping in to see Betty each day and spoke to the nursing staff when he did so. However, he did not appear at any services for several weeks where he had regularly attended before though he seemed friendly enough when the chaplain had encountered him in the lobby of the home once or twice.

JOHN AND MARY

Sr. Helen had a dilemma on her hands at the home where she was the chaplain in charge. The nursing staff or at least one or two of them were expressing concern about the observation that John Henry in the East Wing and a relatively new resident, Mary, were spending a lot of time together and that they were often in his room in the afternoons and early evenings. On one recent occasion, the door to the room had been closed most of the evening and when Nurse Jenny had opened the door to check on John Henry, he and Mary were in bed together albeit on top of the blankets.

Jenny was well aware that cognitively intact residents had rights of privacy. However, she was bothered that Mary clearly had some degree of dementia and that her family had been quite attentive to her upon her admission to the Estates. Jenny doubted that her family would approve of the clear intimacy that was developing. She had scarcely been there four months!! Yet the home had no power to prohibit John Henry from "entertaining" if the two of them wanted to be together and if his "guest" was capable of making a clear decision about such matters. Jenny felt sure that Mary was not so demented as to not know what was going on with John Henry and yet the situation was a concern to her and to staff, especially in terms of how Mary's family would react.

As the weeks passed and the frequent evening liaisons continued, another situation arose. John Henry and Mary expressed the desire to get married. They told Sr. Helen first and asked if she could perform weddings. When she indicated that she was so empowered, they asked her if their families could be part of a small wedding. Had the families been informed of the desire John Henry and Mary had? Well, no, not yet. Anyway, John Henry's attitude was that it wasn't really the business of the families. He and Mary had made up their minds and it was just a matter of setting a date and inviting them to attend. The lack of insight about possible objections from either of their families especially sent a danger signal to Sr. Helen, and she volunteered to help smooth the way for all concerned to be able to consider whether a relationship between John Henry and Mary might be appropriate. She persuaded John Henry and Mary that they needed to allow more time for planning for a wedding and to properly let their families know. Then she was able to bring Mary's family in and to visit with them and with the Administrator of the home about the clearly close relationship between the two residents.

John, Mary and Harry are among the large number of elders who are living longer and longer in varying states of wellness combined with the clear sexual revolution that is encompassing society and raising new pastoral care issues for ministers and chaplains. These include long term survival by dementia and Alzheimer's patients whose spouses are searching for a meaningful way to get on with their lives. Is intimacy allowed or desirable between cognitively impaired marriage partners and their cognitively unimpaired spouses or their non-spouse "friends"? What is the role of an institution in encouraging or discouraging sexual intimacy between persons? How far does the *in loco parentis* role of an institution extend over the lives of older adult residents, both the cognitively impaired and the cognitively intact? What meaningful forms of sexuality are feasible for older widows especially who face living for 10-20 years after the death of a spouse? What concerns should older singles have about sexually transmittable diseases and what precautions should they be encouraged to take? Should there be sex education courses for older adults? These are all potentially issues of concern in pastoral care with older adults.

A growing dilemma faces older adults in today's world. Accepting the messages from media and from years of living that sex is a good, desirable and highly important part of life, older widows especially face limited opportunities to have or share relationships of a sexual nature. Forty-one percent of all women over 65 live alone in the United States, most of whom are widows. In the United States, according to the U.S. Census, there are 75 men for every 100 women 70 to 74 years of age and the number declines to about 50 men for every 100 women ages 80-84. But numbers alone do not tell the whole story. What of the disappointment and despair felt by many older women who find that widowhood offers little chance for times of sharing and affection with a partner, much less of intimacy? What of the loneliness that must grudgingly be accepted when older women face living alone for 10 or 15 or 20 years after losing a spouse? The church and one's family can offer a certain degree of activity and companionship, but are these equal to the closeness of an intimate human bond?

This is a relatively new problem in the aging revolution of our time. In much of the twentieth century, when a couple retired and lived 3-5 years before being separated by the death of one to be typically followed in a short time by the other spouse, sexuality was a limited concern. Today it is. In the past, as older adults progressed in the nightmare of cognitive impairment, he or she contracted other diseases and died. Today, persons like Mary live much longer and thus the number of individuals and families effected by this type of dilemma is greatly increased.

The religious community in Judeo-Christian tradition has always accepted a responsibility for the well-being of its members. Caring for widows and orphans was the role of the temple in Biblical times. We should do no less today. Tracing our sense of the integrity of human life as males and females that the Genesis creation story proclaimed to be "very good" reminds us that human sexuality is a basic quality-of-life issue. The value beyond measure of human life is that all of us are given life by a Creator and sexuality is a major part of that gift of life. Scholars have helped us realize that sex is part of the creative energies of life itself. Libido is basic to the very life force within us. The gift we share, the joy of intimacy with persons, is "very good." In the U.S., the National Council of Churches, the Synagogue Council of America and the U.S. Catholic Conference some time ago joined in affirming this gift of human sexuality. In part they said:

> Human sexuality is a gift of God to be accepted with reverence and joy; . . . It is more than a mechanical instinct. Its many dimensions are intertwined with the total personality and character of the individual. Sex is a dynamic urge or power arising from one's basic maleness or femaleness, and having complex physical, psychological and sexual dimensions. These dimensions, we affirm, must be shaped and guided by spiritual and moral considerations that derive from our Judeo-Christian heritage. Sex education is not, however, only for the young, but is a lifelong task whose aim is to help individuals develop their sexuality in a manner suited to their life stage.[1]

In our secular societies we have allowed the mass media to describe and define meaning in sexuality. As we face challenges to sexual expression in later life, we need to reclaim sex as one of the greatest gifts God gives his people. It is not for any one age group more than another; it is a *gift* from our Creator, *a gift we can all receive and enjoy.*

The centrality of sex for reproduction was understandably a most crucial function of sex for early ages of humanity. Today, however, creation stands in danger of overpopulation and *communion and companionship* rather than procreation are the essential functions of sex and sexuality. Eve and Adam were made for one another's company. While Roman Catholics have emphasized the earlier function of procreation, early Protestants alerted by Rev. Thomas Malthus and his famous theory of population growth versus food production limits were aware of the dangers of run-away population growth and emphasized companionship in marriage.

In current theological reflection, several points need to be stressed in recognizing the role of sex in the lives of older persons. First, companionship, as noted above, is a basic function of intimacy. Second, building upon an incarnational faith, we know that human life for all its frailties is seen as sacred because the body has been a vehicle by which God has come to earth. Christians have been called the "most worldly" of all faith traditions, believing that salvation has become fully human in Jesus Christ. It is reasonable then that human lives are seen as sacred because the incarnation of God's spirit continues in each person born. However, if God is Creator of all life, then human life is not to be taken lightly.

Third, the spirit of God is within OUR LIVES and OUR BODIES suggesting a level of respect and acceptance of our physical natures not widely taught for many generations because of an anti-body pietism in most Christian groups. Such anti-body attitudes trace back to the 'dual-natures' concept of faith rooted in the Greek classic tradition and implanted in New Testament theology by St. Paul in pitting the body against the spirit ("I know that nothing good resides in me, that is, in my physical self." Romans 7:18). That was decidedly NOT a Jewish or Semitic concept of human nature.

Fourth, the doctrines of justification and of grace as a whole among our beliefs are profoundly affected by the understanding of "embodiment" that our faith affirms. If we are justified by grace, and that not of our own doing but a gift of God, if God accepts us through such grace, what exactly is it that is accepted? The Christian ethicist James B. Nelson writes that:

> God's word of acceptance is addressed to the total and sexual self, not simply to a disembodied personality. We might extend Lutheran Theologian, Paul Tillich's language in this manner; you are accepted, the total you. Your body, which you often reject, is accepted by that which is greater than you. Your sexual feelings and unfulfilled yearnings are accepted. You are accepted in your ascetic attempts at self-justification or in your hedonistic alienation from the true meaning of your sexuality. You are accepted in those moments of sexual fantasy which come unbidden and which both delight and disturb you. . . . Simply accept that fact that you are accepted as a sexual person! If that happens to you, you experience grace.[2]

Such acceptance of our lives and bodies as the gift we each have received from God is a profound experience of grace. Freedom to celebrate the feelings and desires of these bodies of ours as normal human aspects of our creation is the opportunity we all have.

Closely akin to self-acceptance is the sense of profound humility. "Authentic humility. . . . is realistic self appreciation."[3] The ability to celebrate sex in later years involves this basic acceptance of the body-self. Nelson describes such an aging experience.

> The physical bodies of most of us fall far short of the ideals portrayed by the advertising industry. Lumpy where they should be slim, skinny where they should be firm, wrinkled where they should be youthful, they are, nevertheless, us, warts and all. And they are graceful bodies because they have been graced.[4]

Such a framework for pastoral care suggests a far more positive and proactive approach to older adult care than comforting persons with the thought that their sexual experiences can be set aside and seen as being all in the past. The National Council of Churches of Christ has said that sex is a powerful urge that must be shaped and guided by spiritual and moral considerations from our Judeo-Christian heritage. To be shaped and guided requires that persons must accept and understand the factors involved and the changes in modern life. Further, this is not a need of children or young adults only but is needed at every stage in life!

If the bodies we have are the heart of God's gift of creation and if God dwells with us, that is, within these bodies, then we can truly help older adults to accept the bodies they have, "warts and all," as God's continuing gift. Pastoral care is intended to help people embrace and celebrate reality, not idealism but the earthy day-by-day reality in which we all live, for THAT is God's daily gift to each of us. Encouraging people to be expressive of their feelings in many ways within the Christian community may be a step toward the embracing of deeper intimate feelings. Fostering openness in warmth, friendship and candor in conversation is a step toward meaningful sexual expression.

To embrace and celebrate our sexual desires and urges is part of that reality also. Too long the church has acted with guilt toward the human body. Too often have we identified the body as the source of sin and not the temple of salvation. Probably this attitude will change far more in the personal affirmation of pastoral care than in bombastic sermons. Pastoral care should help persons to accept and embrace the humanness that is each of us.

Prophetically Barbara P. Payne set out the aging agenda for American churches several years ago in an article in the *Journal of Religion and*

Aging. In an article entitled "Sex and the Elderly: No Laughing Matter in Religion," she noted the major trends in most churches from youth to adult congregations, from male to female participation, and from married to single (or widowed) adults. These, she implied, are the new constituencies. Responses to these changes in congregations should lead to (a) older singles groups for fellowship, (b) support groups for adults following divorce or death of spouse, (c) marital counseling for remarriage families and for later life remarriages, (d) couple groups for older "newlyweds," and (e) marriage revitalization for long-term married couples. She went on to suggest that in the new marriage market of today, there are other choices church members face besides traditional marriage. These include (a) companionship and dating, (b) co-habitation, (c) same-sex relationships, (d) affairs or relationships with married persons or multiple spouses, and (e) no sexual partner (celibacy).[5] Each of these involves a set of yet undefined sexual mores or rules that certainly need to be thought through. Pastoral care and/or counseling can help persons to deal with their unique needs and situations and define what is ethically responsible and sexually satisfactory to them.

Are older persons truly interested in new or continuing sexual activity? A survey contracted by the American Association of Retired Persons in 1999 resoundingly indicated that they are. Conducted by the National Family Research Group in Atlanta of 1384 persons 45 and older, the study found that interest in sex remained active throughout the later adult years.[6] Sex was more vividly of interest for those who had partners and of less interest to those without partners. While perceived state of health and whether their partner was "romantic" influenced men's interest especially, women were affected by whether the partner was understanding and imaginative in sex and also whether women saw themselves as attractive. Nonetheless, the majority saw sex as pleasurable and many saw it as essential to a good relationship.

Given this affirmation of sexual interest, the theological image of sexual embodiment, and given the changing demographics of aging, pastoral care ministries with older adults need to be sensitively and pro-actively dealing with sexual questions and concerns.

CONCLUSION

The first step to addressing the needs for intimacy and sexuality with older adults is to understand that sexuality is a normal part of our human existence. Life is sacred to God and to our faith communities. Sexuality and intimacy are normal parts of life even in the later years. Too often the myth of aging that older adults have no need for or interest in sexuality is embraced by caregivers and they are surprised by situations like the ones Harry, John and Mary present. If we can start from the principles outlined here, then intimacy and sexuality are embraced as a gift of God, not an abnormal act. From this beginning, new solutions to the concerns and interpersonal issues can be constructed.

NOTES

1. Barbara P. Payne "Sex and the Elderly: No Laughing Matter in Religion," *Journal of Religion and Aging* v3, #1/2, (1986): 144.
2. J.B. Nelson, *Embodiment, an Approach to Sexuality and Christian Theology,* Minneapolis: Augsburg Publishing House, 1978, 78-79.
3. Ibid, 82-83.
4. Ibid, 83.
5. Op cit, 145-148.
6. *AARP/Modern Maturity Sexuality Study,* Washington, D.C.: AARP, 1999.

REFERENCES

1999. AARP/Modern Maturity Sexuality Study. Washington, D.C.: AARP.

Nelson, J. B., *Embodiment, an Approach to Sexuality and Christian Theology,* Minneapolis: Augsburg Publishing House, 1978.

Payne, Barbara P., Sex and the Elderly: No Laughing Matter in Religion. *Journal of Religion and Aging,* v.3, #1/2, 1986.

Understanding the Ageing Process:
A Developmental Perspective
of the Psychosocial
and Spiritual Dimensions

Elizabeth MacKinlay, RN, PhD

SUMMARY. This chapter describes a perspective of psychosocial and spiritual development in the later years of life. It outlines a study of nurses conducted in six nursing homes using pre and post workshop tests to identify changes in nurses' assignment of a list of behaviours as psychosocial or spiritual. Use of SPSS found significant changes between the pre and post tests. Pre workshop tests only identified items as spiritual if they included the word God, or Bible. Results from this study highlight the potential role for nurses in aged care to provide spiritual care as part of holistic care. It also highlights the fact that many nurses feel ill prepared for this role. *[Article copies available for a fee from The Haworth Document Delivery Service: 1-800-342-9678. E-mail address: <getinfo@haworthpressinc.com> Website: <http://www.HaworthPress.com> © 2001 by The Haworth Press, Inc. All rights reserved.]*

Rev. Dr. Elizabeth MacKinlay is Senior Lecturer at University of Canberra, Australia, Director of the Centre for Ageing and Pastoral Studies at St. Mark's National Theological Centre, Canberra, and honorary assistant priest at the Anglican Church of the Good Shepherd, ACT.

The second study was supported by the Anglican Diocesan Foundation, Diocese of Canberra and Goulburn and Anglican Retirement Community Services (ARCS) Canberra and Goulburn.

[Haworth co-indexing entry note]: "Understanding the Ageing Process: A Developmental Perspective of the Psychosocial and Spiritual Dimensions." MacKinlay, Elizabeth. Co-published simultaneously in *Journal of Religious Gerontology* (The Haworth Pastoral Press, an imprint of The Haworth Press, Inc.) Vol. 12, No. 3/4, 2001, pp. 111-122; and: *Aging, Spirituality and Pastoral Care: A Multi-National Perspective* (ed: Elizabeth MacKinlay, James W. Ellor, and Stephen Pickard) The Haworth Pastoral Press, an imprint of The Haworth Press, Inc., 2001, pp. 111-122. Single or multiple copies of this article are available for a fee from The Haworth Document Delivery Service [1-800-342-9678, 9:00 a.m. - 5:00 p.m. (EST). E-mail address: getinfo@haworthpressinc.com].

KEYWORDS. Psychosocial development, spiritual development, spiritual integrity, faith development, spiritual behaviours, holistic nursing care

A DEVELOPMENTAL PERSPECTIVE
OF THE PSYCHOSOCIAL AND SPIRITUAL DIMENSIONS

It is often thought that the ageing process is all decline; this certainly appears to be the state from a physiological view. However, and perhaps fortunately, the contribution of the psychosocial and spiritual dimensions of life provides a very different picture of the ageing process. It is far from simple to separate out these two dimensions of ageing; however, it is important to distinguish between these two perspectives when considering the contribution of each to the understanding of the ageing process. This chapter will present a perspective of the ageing process, focusing mainly on spirituality in ageing.

"I'm not really religious." How many times have you heard that said? I asked the 83-year-old woman (I'll call her Eva) what she meant by "being religious"; her response was: "Well going to church and a 'do gooder' but you don't mean it."[1] Often being religious is seen in a negative way that presents a restricted view of the capacity of the human spirit. This was the case for Eva who, despite her claim not to "be religious," had developed a deep sense of spirituality. She had not attended church for many years; she lived alone, in fairly fragile health, surrounded by her cats, her garden, and lots of interesting books. She went to a contact centre for older people each week. Eva had a sense of peace and joy in her life. Eva had grappled with loss and adversity in her long life. She had been both mother and father to her children, as her husband had died while she was pregnant. Eva had never remarried. She had grown spiritually through all of this and continued to question life. Eva described herself as a first World War baby boomer. She said experience had made her question life and its meaning. She was a real survivor and displayed a deep wisdom in the way she spoke of the important things of life.

Some may wonder why I have chosen to use an example of a woman who is not actively involved in church activities, to write of spirituality in ageing. She is one of many I could have chosen, and in a way she is not untypical of many of the older people we meet and care for, or minister to in western society of the early twenty-first century.

In my studies I would have classified Eva as having a sense of spiritual integrity, which I defined as:

> A state where an individual shows by their life example and attitudes, a sense of peace with themselves and others, and development of wholeness of being. The search for meaning and a degree of transcendence is evident.[2]

It seems that what Fowler is describing in his final stage of faith development is spiritual integrity.[3] Spiritual integrity must also be closely related to wisdom; Erikson would say that wisdom is an outcome of ego integrity in ageing.[4] These authors and others have recognised that psychosocial and faith development continues into old age. Indeed, it seems helpful to consider these dimensions from a developmental perspective.

PSYCHOSOCIAL DEVELOPMENT AND AGEING

No consideration of ageing and psychosocial development would be complete without reference to Erikson's eight stages of psychosocial development across the life span. Erikson described the final stage of psychosocial development that occurred in later life as integrity versus despair.[5] It is clear that this stage is not isolated from earlier stages, but is in a sense cumulative. It seems that the individual is able to revisit earlier stages of psychosocial development and attempt to see life experiences in a new way, to reframe what has gone before. There may be tension for an elderly person as they struggle to bring these experiences into a balance. The successful achievement of this leads to integrity, with an outcome of wisdom. However, wisdom itself should be seen as a cumulative process as the person continues to develop psychosocially. This development is frequently witnessed in older people in the naturally occurring process of reminiscence. It seems important in this final life stage to acknowledge recognition of the approaching end of the lifespan. A denial of the inevitability of approaching death may lead to a failure to effectively deal with this stage of psychosocial development.

Peck, recognising the length and complexity of this final stage of psychosocial development, based on Erikson's work, suggested three developmental tasks during the ageing process.[6] Several decades on, these tasks now make even more sense in an ageing society, where people can expect to live for maybe 40-50 years labelled as being 'old.'

Peck called the first task ego differentiation versus work-role preoccupation. This stage involved the role changes, particularly in retirement, that require the individual to make crucial shifts in their personal value system to redefine their worth as older persons. Loss of meaning in life may be a critical factor for older men as they seek to find new meanings in life outside of their work role identity. Rising rates of suicide amongst older men may be a sign of the difficulties that older men face as they age in current western society and struggle to find meaning in later life.[7] This may also become a greater issue for women of the baby boomer generation as work place participation has been both more frequent and longer term for many of these women.

Peck's second task is body transcendence versus body preoccupation. Here the individual has to come to terms with living in an ageing body, accepting that and overcoming problems such as disability and pain that are not uncommonly encountered in chronic illnesses. Successful negotiation of this stage enables the person to transcend the physical decline of the body in ageing. Failure to come to terms with this stage leaves the person preoccupied with the difficulties of the body.

The third task is termed ego-transcendence versus ego preoccupation. Peck saw this as the point of realisation by the person that death would occur to them. Peck saw this task to be letting go of self-centredness and transcending the self. From Frankl's perspective this would be a self-forgetting.[8] These three tasks described by Peck, although described out of a psychosocial view, could quite legitimately be seen from a spiritual perspective as they deal with issues of meaning in life and self-transcendence.

SO WHAT IS SPIRITUALITY?

Still following a developmental approach to understanding ageing, the work of Fowler and others since the early 1980s has added much to understanding faith development across the lifespan.[9,10,11] Although Fowler has used the term 'faith' rather than 'spirituality,' his use of the term is similar. Fowler sees faith as both *relational and as a way of knowing*. It is important to note that Fowler does not state a content of faith; rather he describes a structure of faith development.

Fowler has argued that just as there are stages of psychosocial development across the lifespan, so there are stages of faith development. He describes faith as having seven possible stages (starting at stage 0), but that not everyone will pass through each of these stages.

Older people seem more likely to be at one of the stages from 3 to 6. Stage 3 is called synthetic-conventional faith. This stage is described as everybody's faith, that is conformist in nature. Although this stage is seen as occurring in late childhood, it can also become a terminal stage of faith development for some older adults. The holder of this type is tuned to the expectations and judgments of significant others and has not seen the need to construct his/her own faith stance. It is synthetic in that it lacks analysis and it is accepted without question.

The fourth stage of faith development is termed individuative-reflective faith: In this stage there is a relocation of authority in the self.[12] That is, the individual will be critical of the advice and knowledge of others. This stage is typical in early adulthood, but again, may be a final stage for some. The transition into this stage may occur at any time from young adulthood onwards. Fowler's fifth stage is termed paradoxical-consolidative or conjunctive faith and it is described as a "balanced faith, inclusive faith, a both/and faith."[13] A marked feature of this stage is a "new openness to others and their world views, and a new ability to keep in tension the paradoxes and polarities of faith and life."[14] A new humility and recognition of interdependence is seen at this stage.

The final stage of faith development, called universalising faith, is said to be rare and only occurs in later life. It has been described as a selfless faith; it involves a relinquishing and transcending of the self. Although Fowler's research indicated that few people reached this stage, I would question his findings here and suggest that further research with older adults may show otherwise. I refer particularly to numbers of residents of nursing homes who certainly demonstrate being in this stage of faith development.[15]

Of course we could use the term spirituality rather than faith. I think the term spirituality is the more accessible term, at least in Australian society where spirituality is in more common use in the wider community. The word spirituality is also more widely understood in the health and psychology literature, while it is also in common usage within the fields of pastoral theology and pastoral care.

HOW THEN IS THE SPIRITUAL DIMENSION IN AGEING TO BE UNDERSTOOD?

For older people the real issues of the spiritual dimension may well include worship, but will also include issues of finding ultimate meaning in life, of coping with a failing body, of dealing with loss, and the need for forgiveness and reconciliation. These are all issues belonging to the spiritual domain of life. There is an overlap between psychological and spiritual dimensions, and it seems reasonable to acknowledge this. It may indeed be asked: How important is it to distinguish between psychosocial and spiritual needs? It is suggested that it is important to the extent that *spiritual* needs assessed and diagnosed as *psychosocial* will not be met by appropriate strategies. However, it appears that there is still considerable confusion about what spirituality is both within the community and also amongst health professionals.

SPIRITUALITY IN FRAIL OLDER PEOPLE

I first started listening to the stories of frail older residents of nursing homes in 1992.[16,17] These early studies indicated a range of spiritual need and spiritual well-being amongst the residents. Some older people referred to the nursing home as "God's waiting room." Comments included: "Not even God could help me now I am in a nursing home," "I would rather be dead than here." "I would welcome death." Yet the faith of another older woman allowed her to accept being in a nursing home. These people were residents in well appointed and well maintained nursing homes. These were nursing homes that have prided themselves on the quality of care given to their residents. The context of these comments was a study done in conjunction with a course of continuing education for registered nurses at University of Canberra. One hundred and seventy-two nursing home residents were interviewed by registered nurses in an assessment of spiritual needs of older people. In this study the nurses reported that they benefited greatly from the experience of this study, one saying: . . . "what an important area this is for registered nurses . . . we do not properly address this area." They were often surprised at how ready the residents were to share their concerns, and that for a number of residents, it was the first time they had felt free to talk about the deeper things of life. These nurses learnt a lot about the people they had cared for, for months, or years. These were things that led them to see nursing in a new way, and to change the way they were giving care.

A STUDY OF SPIRITUAL AWARENESS
OF REGISTERED NURSES WORKING IN NURSING HOMES

These same nurses initiated the request for a project to raise nurse awareness of the spiritual needs of older adult residents in nursing homes. This request coincided with my concerns at the lack of spiritual care residents in nursing homes were receiving. Thus the project to raise nurse awareness of their own spirituality and assist them to recognise spiritual needs of their residents in six nursing homes (five in Canberra and one in New South Wales) was developed. The study consisted of a pre-test, that examined nurse understanding of the term spirituality, and also asked them to identify a number of behaviours as being in the physical, psychosocial or spiritual domains, or a combination of psychosocial and spiritual (see Table 1). The subsequent analysis, using SPSS was set up to take account of moves from psychosocial to spiritual or the reverse.

A workshop followed where nurses examined their individual spirituality and how this impacted on their own lives. Following this, basic strategies were outlined to enable the workshop participants to identity spiritual needs in residents and either meet these, or refer residents to appropriate pastoral care providers. A post-test was administered after the workshops.

COMPARISON OF THE PRE AND POST CONTINUING EDUCATION SURVEYS

Each item was compared, before and after the session, the sample size for each item varied from 35 to 53.

The objective of analysis was to determine whether there was a change in the respondent's perceptions of the spiritual aspect of each activity on the inventory between the pre and post session surveys. All post session surveys were completed less than two weeks after the education sessions. Follow up of some respondents was difficult, due to people going on leave, or being unobtainable for other reasons.

Significant changes in participant identification of the spiritual dimension were shown between the pre and post surveys (Table 2). In the pre session inventory, the only items which were rated high as spiritual behaviours were those associated with worship, or that contained the word "God" or "Bible." This is consistent with a common perception that religion and spirituality are synonymous, yet human spirituality is a much broader dimension than that. Comparing the pre and post response, the change was for more respondents to identify the spiritual dimension, either alone, or with the psychosocial dimension.

These nurses subsequently identified the spiritual dimension more frequently in their work with older nursing home residents. In fact one

TABLE 1. List of spiritual behaviours/actions developed for the study

1. Praying with patient 2. Assisting a person to find meaning in suffering and death 3. Listening to a patient 4. Supporting a person in their hope of life after death 5. Developing a trusting relationship with patient 6. Reading the Bible or other religious material 7. Calling the chaplain or minister 8. Facilitating reminiscence 9. Assisting an elderly person to find meaning in life 10. Caring with integrity for an elderly person 11. Assisting a person in the process of dying 12. Facilitating relationship with an elderly person	13. Assisting an elderly person to worship according to their faith 14. Assisting an elderly person who is fearful of their future 15. Supporting a person in their feeling of being loved by others/God 16. Assisting a person to deal with feelings of guilt 17. Caring for a person who feels hopeless 18. Referral of a person who needs forgiveness 19. Facilitating reconciliation among family members 20. Facilitating reconciliation with God 21. Assisting a person to achieve a sense of self-acceptance 22. Honouring a person's integrity 23. Assisting a person to deal with anger 24. Assisting a person to deal with grief

problem that emerged for me following this study was receiving more referrals from nursing staff for cases of spiritual distress/need than I could meet. Nurses who have completed studies in spirituality and nursing could address a number of these issues as part of their holistic nursing care.[18] It was evident that many of the nurses working in the nursing homes where these studies were conducted had no preparation in providing spiritual care, and did not feel comfortable providing this care. While my sessions with them certainly increased their sensitivity to the spiritual needs of their residents, it did not provide them with strategies they felt comfortable to use.

AN UNDERSTANDING OF SPIRITUALITY

For an adequate understanding of spirituality it is necessary to consider: First, the human need for ultimate meaning in each person, whether this is fulfilled through relationship with God, or some sense of 'other'; or whether some other sense of meaning becomes the guiding force within the individual's life. Second, human spirituality involves relationship with others. Spirituality is a part of every human being. Once acknowledging the universal nature of human spirituality, there is a real need to have a definition of spirituality that is inclusive of all religious groups and of the secular.

TABLE 2. Using McNemar's test, at the 95% level of significance, 10 items were significant (Chi sq (1 df) critical value at 95% 3.84)

Item	Behaviour	Score
3	listening to a patient	6.23
8	facilitating reminiscence	4.76
11	assisting a person in the process of dying	6.00
14	assisting an elderly person who is fearful of their future	9.00
15	supporting a person in their feeling of being loved by others/God	4.50
16	assisting a person to deal with feelings of guilt	11.27
17	caring for a person who feels hopeless	4.45
19	facilitating reconciliation among family members	8.89
22	honouring a person's integrity	7.36
23	assisting a person to deal with anger	8.07

It seems appropriate to consider spirituality as having two components, a broad, generic component and a specific component. The generic component is that which lies at the core of each human's being. It is that which searches and yearns for relationship in life and for meaning in existence. Individual humans may find this need addressed in all sorts of situations in life, in love, in joy, in suffering and in pain and loss. Ashbrook says: "Beyond the self of culture lies the soul in God, the core of each person's being."[19] The specific component of spirituality is understood as the way each individual works out their spirituality in their lives. This may be in the practice of a particular religion, it may be through relationship with other people and in community, work, or through particular centres of meaning and interests in life.

A DEFINITION OF SPIRITUALITY

There are many definitions of spirituality. The operational definition used in my studies takes into account the main characteristics of the sample of older people interviewed. These were Christians and others who acknowledged no faith or denominational affiliation. This definition of spirituality was:

That which lies at the core of each person's being, an essential dimension which brings meaning to life. Constituted not only by religious practices, but understood more broadly, as relationship with God, however God or ultimate meaning is perceived by the person, and in relationship with other people.[20]

WHAT HAPPENS WITH SPIRITUALITY IN THE AGEING PROCESS?

As the person reaches and passes middle age there is a tendency to become more introspective and to come to a new sense of time. Neugarten, taking a psychological perspective, sees this as a refocus from time yet to live, to time already lived.[21] Reminiscence becomes more important, and is now well recognised as a spiritual task of ageing. As individuals become more conscious of the approaching end of their lives the search for final meaning of life gains greater urgency. Questions such as "Why was I here?" "Has my life been worthwhile?" gain a new importance.

A number of authors have recognised changes that occur in the spiritual dimension in ageing. Clements[22] writes of spiritual development being the developmental stage of the fourth quarter of life, Fischer writes of the necessity of letting go to be able to move onward, viewing this as the ability to affirm life in the face of death.[23] Frankl wrote of the search for final meanings in life, as one grows older. [24] Kimble too writes of the search for meaning in later life and the spiritual nature of this search.[25]

The losses of loved ones and the losses of roles of middle life may lead to a new questioning of life and its meaning. In conjunction with this, the onset of chronic illnesses and disabilities, and the physical decline so commonly encountered in ageing lead to a shift in focus from doing to being. This may be used as an opportunity to reflect and become more introspective, or it may become a time of struggle and tension in the process of wanting to hold onto a mid-life focus of associating meaning in life through roles and activities in life. In a sense there is an inextricable connection between physical decline and spiritual development. It seems that in ageing, as Paul wrote: 2 Corinthians 4:16: "Even though our outer nature is wasting away, our inner nature is being renewed day by day." Transcendence and growing into a sense of integrity as well as coming to final meanings of life can be seen as critical tasks of ageing. There is the potential for spiritual development to continue to the point of death. In fact it can be said that the process of dying itself is part of the spiritual journey.

CONCLUSION

This chapter has examined ageing taking a developmental perspective, considering this under two related aspects, psychosocial developmental processes and spiritual developmental processes. While there are close links, and in fact, interactions between the two aspects, there are also differences that are important to acknowledge. When the developmental aspects of ageing are too narrowly defined in terms of the psychosocial, one result is that access is denied to spiritual interventions of the Sacraments, and pastoral care. The risks of assigning all things to the spiritual domain has the disadvantage of denying access to the rich strategies of the psychosocial domain that are also valuable in assisting older people to continue to develop in these dimensions in later life. A better understanding of the spiritual dimension in ageing seems an important avenue to explore in examining the holistic role for nurses as well as the roles of other health professionals and clergy.

NOTES

1. E.B. MacKinlay, "The Spiritual Dimension of Ageing: Meaning in Life, Response to Meaning, and Well Being in Ageing" (doctoral thesis, LaTrobe University, 1998).

2. Ibid., 292.

3. J.W. Fowler, *Stages of Faith: The Psychology of Human Development and the Quest for Meaning* (San Francisco: Harper, 1981).

4. E.H Erikson, J.M. Erikson, and H.Q. Kivnick, *Vital Involvement in Old Age* (New York: W.W. Norton & Co, 1986).

5. Ibid.

6. R.C. Peck, "Psychological development in the second half of life," in *Middle Age and Aging: A Reader in Social Psychology,* edited by B.L. Neugarten (Chicago: The University of Chicago Press, 1968).

7. R. Hassan, *Suicide Explained: The Australian Experience* (Melbourne: Melbourne University Press, 1995).

8. V.E. Frankl, *Man's Search for Meaning* (New York: Washington Square Press, 1984).

9. J.W. Fowler, 1981.

10. J.W. Fowler, K.E. Nipkow, F. Schweitzer, eds., *Stages of Faith and Religious Development: Implications for Church, Education, and Society* (London: SCM Press Ltd., 1992).

11. J.W. Fowler in *Faith Development and Fowler,* edited by C. Dykstra and S. Parks (Birmingham, Alabama: Religious Education Press, 1986).

12. Fowler, *Stages of Faith,* 179.

13. J. Astley, L.J. Francis, *Christian Perspectives on Faith Development* (Grand Rapids: William B. Eerdmans Publishing Company, 1992), viii.

14. Ibid., xxii.

15. E.B. MacKinlay, Data from study of elderly residents of nursing homes in Canberra, Australia (Unpublished. Study completed 2000).

16. E.B. MacKinlay, "Spiritual Needs of the Elderly Residents of Nursing Homes" (Unpublished report, submitted in part fulfillment of requirements for BTh at St Mark's National Theological Centre, Canberra, 1992).

17. E.B. MacKinlay, "Spirituality and Ageing: Bringing Meaning to Life," in *St Mark's Review*, Spring 155 (1993), 26-30.

18. E.B. MacKinlay, "Ageing, spirituality and the nursing role," in *Spirituality: The Heart of Nursing*, edited by S. Ronaldson (Melbourne: AUSMED Publications, 1997).

19. J.B. Ashbrook, *Minding the Soul: Pastoral Counseling as Remembering* (Minneapolis: Fortress Press, 1996), 74.

20. MacKinlay, "Spiritual Needs of the Elderly Residents."

21. B.L. Neugarten, "Adult personality: Towards a psychology of the life cycle," in *Middle Age and Aging: A Reader in Social Psychology*, edited by B.L. Neugarten (Chicago: The University of Chicago Press, 1968).

22. W.M. Clements, "Spiritual development in the fourth quarter of life," in *Spiritual Maturity in the Later Years*, edited by J.J. Seeber (New York: The Haworth Press, Inc., 1990), 69.

23. K. Fischer, *Winter Grace: Spirituality for the Later Years* (New York: Paulist Press, 1985).

24. Frankl, *Man's Search for Meaning.*

25. M.A. Kimble, S.H. McFadden, J. W. Ellor, and J.J. Seeber, eds., *Aging, Spirituality, and Religion: A Handbook* (Minneapolis: Augsburg Fortress Press, 1995).

Through a Glass Darkly:
A Dialogue Between Dementia and Faith

Malcolm Goldsmith, MSc, BSocSc

SUMMARY. Our understanding and experience of dementia is changing and developing, as is our understanding and experience of faith. Both
areas offer signs of hope but both also contain evidence of discrimination
and disenchantment. This paper seeks to explore these parallel worlds
from the perspective of the person with dementia, the family carer, the
institutional carer and the community of faith. It closes with a challenge
to theology to demonstrate just what is the Good News of the Gospel for
the person with dementia. *[Article copies available for a fee from The
Haworth Document Delivery Service: 1-800-342-9678. E-mail address:
<getinfo@haworthpressinc.com> Website: <http://www.HaworthPress.com>
© 2001 by The Haworth Press, Inc. All rights reserved.]*

KEYWORDS. Dementia, faith, carers (family and institutional), theology, hope

Malcolm Goldsmith is a priest in the Scottish Episcopal Church and Rector of St.
Cuthbert's Church in Colinton, Edinburgh and is formerly a Research Fellow with the
Dementia Services Development Centre in the University of Stirling.

Address correspondence to: Malcolm Goldsmith, 6 Westgarth Avenue, Colinton,
Edinburgh EH13 0BD Scotland (E-mail: Malcolm.Goldsmith@btinternet.com).

I am taking *Faith* to mean the practice, the theory and the experience of being a disciple
of Jesus. It therefore breathes life into the word *Religion,* but is more specific and rooted
than the word *Spirituality.*

This paper was presented to the *Ageing, Spirituality and Pastoral Care in the 21st Century* in Canberra Australia, January 2000, and subsequently amended for publication.

[Haworth co-indexing entry note]: "Through a Glass Darkly: A Dialogue Between Dementia and Faith."
Goldsmith, Malcolm. Co-published simultaneously in *Journal of Religious Gerontology* (The Haworth
Pastoral Press, an imprint of The Haworth Press, Inc.) Vol. 12, No. 3/4, 2001, pp. 123-138; and: *Aging, Spirituality and Pastoral Care: A Multi-National Perspective* (ed: Elizabeth MacKinlay, James W. Ellor, and Stephen Pickard) The Haworth Pastoral Press, an imprint of The Haworth Press, Inc., 2001, pp. 123-138. Single
or multiple copies of this article are available for a fee from The Haworth Document Delivery Service
[1-800-342-9678, 9:00 a.m. - 5:00 p.m. (EST). E-mail address: getinfo@haworthpressinc.com].

A few years ago, before the BBC went 'high-tec' there used to be a sequence before the news programmes which showed two globes, of differing projections, each turning at a different speed and, as it were, interacting with each other–in much the same way that a large cog engages with a small cog as they both revolve. I want to suggest that the differing worlds of dementia and faith, which each have their own internal cohesion, concerns and organic life, can also engage with each other. It is my contention that in that process of engagement each can be significantly affected by their contact with the other.

Let me stay with that BBC image for a moment, and suggest that one of those globes is the world of dementia. It is a changing world, and like a globe it revolves on its axis as it moves through time and space. It is changing both in the way that dementia is experienced and perceived and also in the way that services respond to and support people with dementia. The world of dementia and of dementia care is a world of change, with wide extremes. Within the turbulence of those changes we can discover wonderful examples of heroic living and imaginative care, and–sadly–we can also discover the ghastly edges of discrimination, punitive care and 'warehousing' in an impoverished system.

The second of my two globes is the world of faith. This also is a changing world. There are changes in the way that faith is experienced and perceived, and in the way that faith is articulated, described, presented and experienced. It also is a world of change with wide extremes. Within the turbulence of those changes too we can discover wonderful examples of heroic living and–sadly–we can also discover the ghastly edges of discrimination, punitive approaches and unimaginative systems.

There is a form of dementia understanding that is strictly biomedical and which is highly structured, authoritarian and, from my perspective, closed in its approach. As I see it, this approach is at best responsible and deeply committed, but at worst it is dehumanising because it treats people as objects, regarding the disease, not the person, as the principal point of interest. Similarly there is a form of religious expression that is highly structured, authoritarian and closed in its approach. At its best it is highly systematic and contains an inbuilt consistency, but at worst it is dehumanising because it treats people as objects, regarding the theological structure or doctrinal 'soundness' as the principal point of concern. There are also forms of dementia care which are liberating, innovative, caring, costly, vulnerable and precious; and precisely the same thing can be said about some expressions of faith.

It is my conviction that the worlds of dementia and of faith can dialogue with each other. In fact, they need to dialogue with each other. Now the very nature of dialogue is that each side listens to the other and responds in the light of what the other has said or done, and as that response is made, so the conditions are changed and they continue to change as the dialogue continues. Breakdown occurs when one or both of the parties fails to listen and fails to respond creatively, preferring to protect a set position and demanding that the other be 'colonised.'

At the heart of the new approach in dementia care is the insistence on placing the person with dementia at the centre, and honouring them and listening to their voice, difficult though it may be to hear that voice. There is a new culture emerging in dementia care; slowly, partial, fragmentary–to be found in one place but not in another. It is an approach which, whilst being totally honest about the devastating effects of the illnesses which underline dementia, also focuses upon the positive and emphasises what can still be done, and which refuses to write off people because of what they say or do. It is an approach which accepts behaviour, utterances and confusions and which strives constantly to enhance and enfold people with dementia with care and concern, with respect and (dare I say it) with reverence.

I am well aware of how difficult this is for many people. I know of carers stressed-out to the point of breakdown. I know many institutions lack the resources to care in ways that they would like to whilst others lack the imagination or the skills to provide care of the highest quality. Dementia care is in a state of flux. It is a mixture of the imaginatively committed and the frankly awful, and too often it is a lottery as to which sort of care a person receives.

To provide imaginative care of the highest quality is a daunting task. It is often lonely and it often seems as if we go two steps backward for every one step forward. There are strong temptations to 'batten down the hatches,' to opt for the lines of least resistance and to lose hope, overwhelmed by the difficulty of the task. Creative dementia care is a perilous journey for the carer, a journey of faith, hope and charity and there is a desperate need for encouragement, for hope, for conversations and for people to laugh and cry with. The world of dementia care can be a lonely world–a journey through a valley of the shadow of death. And yet there are signs of change, signs of hope. This is how Tom Kitwood summed up the situation towards the end of the book which was published shortly before his untimely death:

> In the radical reconsideration of dementia . . . almost every cherished assumption has now been called into question. Even the category of 'organic mental disorder' which has underpinned a century or more of psychiatric practice has not stood up well to the test of time. Among the changes that have occurred, one fact stands out above all others. It is that men and women who have dementia have emerged from the places where they were hidden away; they have walked onto the stage of history and begun to be regarded as persons in the full sense. Dementia, as a concept, is losing its terrifying associations with the raving lunatic in the old time asylum. It is being perceived as an understandable human condition, and those who are affected by it have begun to be recognised, welcomed, embraced and heard. The achievements of biomedical science, although much vaunted in the media, are insignificant in comparison to this quiet revolution.[1]

Now let me return to the sphere of faith. In a world of conflicting and competing ideologies, as secularisation and secularism take root in our communities, many churches and faith communities often feel themselves to be under threat. They can so easily adopt a laager-mentality and feel that they must protect themselves against adversaries attacking them from all sides. If the threats that I have already mentioned are not enough they also strive to fend off radicalism, liberalism, universalism and syncretism–and these are merely the enemies from within! There is an approach to faith which is deeply suspicious of change and which is so obsessed by the sin and unbelief that it sees all around that it fears–it fears for itself, it fears for the church and ultimately it fears for God. It is caught up in the same journey of disintegration that is sometimes seen to be the inevitable outcome of dementia. It is ultimately a journey towards death. Not death with a sense of completion and satisfaction but death involving bewilderment and estrangement; not a death accompanied by faith but, paradoxically, the death of faith. There exists, within many communities of faith, a sort of fatalistic acceptance of marginalisation, of irrelevance, of confusion and of decline and death. We might call it *'the dementia of dogma underpinned by a theology of despair.'*

But there is also, sometimes interwoven with this and sometimes discovered quite separately from it, a theology of life; an experience of a journey of faith which is excited and thrilled by the very precariousness and vulnerability of its practice. The signs of hope which can be seen in the new culture of dementia care have parallels in experiences of faith which emerge in similar situations of apparent decline and disintegration. I am excited by and confident about the ways in which the world of faith and the world of dementia can dialogue with, and learn, from each other.

The possibility of there being such common ground between faith and dementia came to me quite suddenly several years ago when reading a poem by the Welsh priest R.S. Thomas. The poem is about God but it seemed to me that it could also have been about a person with dementia.

> *You show me two faces*
> *that of a flower opening*
> *and of a fist contracting*
> *like the gripping of ice.*
>
> *You speak to me with two*
> *voices, one thundering*
> *on the ear's drum, the other*
> *one mistakable for silence.*
>
> *Father, I said, domesticating*
> *an enigma; and as though*
> *to humour me you came.*
> *But there are precipices*
>
> *within you. Mild and dire,*
> *now and absent, like us but*
> *wholly other-which side*
> *of you am I to believe?* [2]

(Printed with permission)

The question to God, and also to the person with dementia is "Which side of you am I to believe?" Of course the answer is both sides, and it is this living with paradox, with contradictions and ambiguity which is so difficult.

In another poem R.S. Thomas writes about the hidden-ness of God, a theme which seems to resonate with the experience of many carers:

> *It is this great absence*
> *that is like a presence, that compels*
> *me to address it without hope*
> *of a reply. It is a room I enter*
> *from which someone has just gone* [3]

(Printed with permission)

This experience of absence is by no means the whole story. Increasingly ways are being found of communicating with people with dementia so that it is not always the case that we address someone "without hope of a reply," and this is one of the characteristics of the new climate or culture of dementia care. Similarly with faith–there are ways of growing in faith which take on board a context in which the experience of God is not always immediate and where the apparent absence of God can itself be the raw material for growth and discipleship.

I read recently that we are often frightened by mysteries and to deal with this fear we convert mysteries into problems because we can control problems.[4] Dementia is still a mystery to most of us; we neither understand where it has come from and we are fearful of where it will lead. This chapter begins to open up the dialogue between dementia and faith from five different perspectives firstly from the position of the person with dementia; secondly from the standpoint of the family carer, then thirdly, from the standpoint of the institutional carer; fourthly from the position of the local community of faith and fifthly and finally from the perspective of theology.

THE PERSON WITH DEMENTIA

For the person with dementia this is a journey into the unknown. We are now, at last beginning to get some records from people themselves rather than from observers and what is clear is that people with dementia do not all experience it in the same way. For all of them it is an illness, and it is a progressive and bewildering illness, but people are affected in different ways and we are told very little when we are told that Bill or Susan has Alzheimer's Disease. The person's personality, their general health and sense of well-being, their interests, their social and family relationships, their capacity to change or to cope with change, their observational patterns and their relationship with reality, built up over the years, all combine to play their part in determining how they will manage and cope with this new stage in their life.

We know that very few people are given a sufficiently early diagnosis in order that they might have the opportunity to talk about their illness or the time and resources to plan for it. People with dementia will mostly have been protected (though that is hardly the appropriate word) by a process of denial and collusion by their friends and family, so that they slowly enter into the world of dementia without having had much mental, emotional or spiritual preparation for it. There is then a tendency for them to be marginalised and either by choice or by circumstance they often find themselves left out of conversations, planning or general activities. They may therefore retreat into silence or depression, or they may come out fighting. But whatever their response there is the likelihood that it will be interpreted as being 'a problem.' Kitwood has identified a whole range of experiences which make up what he has described as 'malignant social psychology.' They are:

treachery; disempowerment; infantilization; intimidation; labelling; stigmatisation; outpacing; invalidation; banishment; and objectification.

Then to this original list of ten he later added

ignoring; imposition; withholding; accusation; disruption; mockery and disparagement [5]

From the perspective of faith, surely here is an example of the suffering servant, the least of his brethren, reminding us that what we did for them we did also for him; I am reminded of Psalm 22 every time I reflect upon Kitwood's malignant social psychology.

My God, my God, look upon me; why hast thou forsaken me;
and art so far from my health, and from the words of my complaint.
O my God, I cry in the day-time, but thou hearest not;
and in the night-season also I take no rest. . . .
But as for me, I am a worm, and no man:
a very scorn of men, and the outcast of the people.
All they that see me laugh me to scorn;
they shoot out their lips and shake their heads . . .

O go not from me for trouble is hard at hand;
and there is none to help me.
Many oxen are come about me;
fat bulls of Basan close me in on every side.
They gape upon me with their mouths:
as it were a ramping and a roaring lion.
I am poured out like water, and all my bones are out of joint:
my heart also in the midst of my body is even like melting wax.
My strength is dried up like a potsherd, and my tongue cleaveth to my
  gums:
and thou shalt bring me into the dust of death . . .
But be not thou far from me O Lord:
thou art my succour, haste thee to help me[6]

And what are the spiritual needs of the person with dementia? Surely
to be accepted, to be given worth and honour, to be befriended and to be
listened to, to be placed within a wider context of peace and security, of
beauty and of love. They are the needs of all who are human, but with an
extra dimension of sensitivity because people with dementia are especially vulnerable; they may be lonely and bewildered, they may be
grieving and desperately trying to communicate, they are almost certainly frightened at some stage in their illness. They may need to be re-
assured by hearing the old stories told to them again, to be reminded of
the great myths and tales of their culture, to hear again the music and to
see the signs and the symbols which have sustained them through the
years. Since when has a failure to articulate need meant that there was
no need? Since when has a position on the edge meant that the person
was less needy than one situated near the centre? Since when has not
having a memory of past nourishment negated the need for present
feeding?
    The person with dementia presents a challenge to the community of
faith. A challenge to be accepted unconditionally, to be valued and hon-
oured, to be treated with respect and dignity and to be recognised as a
child of God, loved, welcomed, forgiven and recognised as a brother or
sister, and to be fed. But more than that, to be discovered as being a vehicle or a channel for the love of God to others, for it may well be that
God chooses to reveal the very heart of the mystery of life and of love
through the vulnerability of the person from whom pride and pretence
has been stripped away.

The full range of spiritual resources must be available and accessible to the person with dementia so that they can say alongside Dag Hammarskjold

Night is drawing nigh
For all that has been–Thanks
To all that shall be–yes! [7]

THE FAMILY CARER

If every person who has dementia is different, so is every family and so are the responses that they make. John Bayley's tender little book "Iris: A memoir of Iris Murdoch" [8] about his novelist wife, has some telling insights;

> One needs very much to feel that the unique individuality of one's spouse has not been lost in the common symptoms of a clinical condition (p. 42) . . . and . . . our mode of communication seems like underwater sonar, each bouncing pulsations off the other, and listening for an echo. The baffling moments at which I cannot understand what Iris is saying, or about whom or what–moments which can promote anxieties, though never, thank goodness, the raging frustration typical of many Alzheimer's sufferers–can sometimes be dispelled by embarking on a joky parody of helplessness, and trying to make it mutual. Both of us at a loss for words (p. 44) . . . and . . . Alzheimer's, which can accentuate personality traits to the point of demonic parody, has only been able to exaggerate a natural goodness in her. (p. 59)

Bayley's experience contrasts starkly with that of the journalist Linda Grant who wrote about her mother in a book full of frustration and anger.[9], I will give you three quotes:

> One of Multi-Infarct Dementia's cruellest tricks is to preserve in its victim until quite a late stage, some insight into what is going on in their mind, so that they can observe themselves lose their own sanity. Depression and emotional instability is a marked characteristic of this disease and who wouldn't be miserable watching themselves go mad. (p. 129)

The dogma is this: Social Services comply with what the elderly client wants. What does my mother want? It depends on which sense of herself is in the ascendant at any given moment and with each of these there is no memory of there being another self that wanted something else. What does the self I had come across crying on the toilet want? (p. 179)

But she is so angry, so aggressive–she took me by the shoulders and pushed me out of the room, once, when I told her I didn't have the time to take her out. What Michele and I are after is a chemical solution. How about Prozac, the happy drug? (p. 235)

It does not behove us to make any judgement on those extracts for none of us knows how we would react in her circumstances, and therefore one of the first things we must learn when meeting the carers of people with dementia is tolerance, forbearance and a deep sense of respect. These are the people who have had to discover ways of coping creatively and courageously with a situation that nothing could have prepared them for. Imagine what the writer of this poem might have had to cope with

> *In the end my mother lay*
> *body-bound, curled like a foetus*
> *fretting for a peppermint, a sip of whiskey,*
> *the pillow turned this way and that*
> *and she a woman who, buoyant in silk*
> *and shingled hair, stood on the hill*
> *at Fiesole reciting her Browning to the wind* [10]

(Permission to print)

These are people who have cried enough tears to fill a well; they are people who have experienced a lifetime's emotions in the space of a few months or years, and who ask themselves over and over again, "How can we sing the Lord's song in a strange land?" Here are people hungering and thirsting for a word of hope, for a sense of meaning and who are often wracked by a deep sense of guilt. David Keck has observed, "one of the harder lessons of caregiving is that we must be humble and aspire to be stewards not saviours."[11] The challenge to faith must be obvious, but what does the community of faith learn from an encounter with carers? One thing is certain, they need to hear and hear time and time again the words of Vaclav Havel, the Czech dramatist, philosopher and statesman, *Hope is not about believing you can change things. Hope is about believing you make a difference.*

People can and do make a difference, and the difference can have a profound effect upon the person who has dementia, and also upon the general environment in which they all live. And this is Gospel stuff! We are talking here neither about miraculous healing nor about heroic suffering, but about discovering a new way of thinking and a new way of being. Kitwood, reflecting on his earliest encounters with dementia said that he was "seduced by the prevailing view–(that) dementia (was) a death that leaves the body behind." He was to discover and commit the rest of his life to exploring and proclaiming the sense of worth and dignity and purpose in the experience of dementia. A view that turns the accepted ways of looking at things upside down–now where have I come across that idea before?

THE INSTITUTIONAL CARER

If people really can make a difference, then there are opportunities unbounded in our nursing homes, residential homes and hospitals for really creative work to be done and for Gospel qualities of care and understanding to be demonstrated. A person in my own congregation who has been in severe decline for the past nine to twelve months and who has been testing her family's compassion and tolerance to the limit has recently been admitted to hospital for reasons unrelated to her dementia. There, in a different context, indeed she believes herself to be a in five star hotel, she has found new purpose and a new zest for life. Her confusion and her dementing illness still progress, but in a different context and with skilled care she demonstrates the fact that admission into residential or institutional care need not been seen as family failure nor as one more regressive step, but it may open up new possibilities, new horizons. I cannot emphasise too strongly the wonderful and unique opportunities that present themselves to staff in these places.

I remember, in a different context, twenty plus years ago visiting my mother in hospital and learning that the evening before she had been told that in order to stop the spread of a facial cancer she must have her nose amputated. It was a student nurse who sat by her bedside through the lonely hours of that night bringing her comfort and courage. God can work through the most unassuming people in the most unexpected ways, and this is certainly true of dementia care.

I cut my theological teeth in the 1960s; they were wonderful days with intellectual curiosity being joined to social commitment and the motif of Martin Luther King's *I Have a Dream* underpinning so much of our study and our action. And now forty years later, I have this new dream. It is a dream of a people marginalised by illness and discriminated against by powerlessness being moved to centre stage to remind us that vulnerability is of the very essence of the Gospel and that time and time again God speaks to us through those who have no voice, or whose words come to us as metaphors–so easily tossed aside and yet demanding to be heard. Listen to the voice of this lady whose frustrations and experience of impotence have been captured by my colleague John Killick, a writer and a poet who has spent the last seven or eight years talking with people with dementia and recording those conversations. The speaker in this poem, 'The Monkey Puzzle,' feels that everything about her existence has become 'managed' without consultation.

I'm suffering from the Monkey Puzzle.
The Monkey Puzzle is this place.
The puzzle is how to cope with the Monkeys.
I can't remember anything of today
Except the peppering of my tongue. Yes,
My mouth was peppered again this morning.
I believe it is part of the Monkey Puzzle.
These little Monkeys have two legs,
You know, and wear suits.
These whiskers that are growing
around the lower part of my face,
I did think they formed a part
of the category of the Monkey Puzzle,
put there to irritate newcomers.

I've come to the conclusion
that what we should do
is educate these Monkeys.
We should make it perfectly clear
that there are certain things
that are not done, even though
I know that they are laughing
their heads off behind my back.

People are pushing things down my neck
I don't believe its even for a joke–
It's pure badness. Next time anybody says
'Put that in your mouth!' I'll take a flying leap
and punch them. It's an unignorable fact
that they are mucking me about.

If this is another bit of the Monkey Puzzle,
then Monkey will know what it's got!
I'll run amok a-shutter, I really will,
I'll just go wild and frighten them[12]

(Permission to print)

It is in places such as this that the practical outworking of the Gospel takes root. People of faith stand on the conviction that there is no place where God's Spirit cannot enter with transforming and transfiguring power, and that there is no person beyond the scope of God's mercy and compassion. This is surely good news for the person with dementia and the ministers of that news are often the poorest paid in our community and have some of the most menial tasks to do.

Who are you–walking to the toilet every few minutes? Who are you–wiping bottoms, answering the same question time and time again, sitting with those who weep and absorbing the anger and the frustration of those who do not know where they are?

Who am I? I am a minister of the Gospel of love, and this angry lady is my sister and this weeping man my brother.

THE COMMUNITY OF FAITH

I recently read the Newsletter of a group working with people with learning disabilities. It quoted that passage from 1Corinthians 12(v22) "On the contrary, those parts of the body that seem to be weaker are indispensable" and went on to say "this verse says that such people are indispensable, we cannot do without them and the church is incomplete without them. I would go so far as to say that until a church is ready to welcome and integrate people with learning disabilities into its fellowship it will be impoverished." And surely the same is true for people with dementia. But note, the prime motivation is not for our own heath and wellbeing but for theirs.

I know it is not easy. People with dementia so easily can become invisible to the church, and slowly their carers may also become invisible–they slowly fade away. I look back with shame on my five years as a Rector of a busy church in the centre of an English city some twenty years ago. I don't think I can recall meeting a single person with dementia during that period. You see, if you don't look for them and if you are not ready to welcome and accept them, then they so easily go elsewhere–and in terms of the church that 'elsewhere' invariably becomes 'nowhere'–and we are all impoverished as a result, all of us.

In my present parish I find it a constant challenge to integrate and honour people with dementia and I am both moved and humbled by the ways in which members of the congregation go out of their way to befriend and stand alongside them. People with dementia can come amongst us as angels in disguise; we can learn from them, we can receive from them and we can share so much with them. But they are also a constant challenge, testing our capacity to welcome, requiring us to be more accessible and tolerant and reminding us week-by-week and day-by-day that we are knit together in an invisible fellowship of common humanity. They also challenge our theological assumptions and force us to ask questions–not so much about them as about ourselves. Are we really a community of faith, a community of love, a community of forgiveness? The answer of course is both yes and no–we do believe, but help thou our unbelief; we do love, but so often we pick and choose whom we love and we have not yet reached a level of indiscriminate and reckless loving, and yes we do try to forgive because we know how much we too need to be forgiven.

The presence of people with dementia in our midst reminds us of the importance of symbolism and ritual. They challenge our reliance upon words and words and yet even more words. They point to the need to look again at the ways in which we try and so often fail to communicate–most especially in listening. With a little time and imagination it is possible for us to reflect on what we might do for them, but the bigger question is to reflect upon what we might learn from them and in what ways they might contribute to our common life. Whilst all the time being aware of the fact that these people are suffering from a most awful illness, and it is sometimes quite difficult–in fact it is very difficult sometimes–to remember that when we are hard pressed and short of time. In such times it is we who need to fall back upon the unsearchable riches of God to discover once again that divine grace which is all-sufficient.

THE CHALLENGE TO THEOLOGY

I am writing here as a Christian; I suspect though that these or similar sentiments are relevant to other faiths or value systems.

So much of our theology is built upon a structure of belief, penitence and faith. We have a historic faith, we require understanding and we require personal conviction and personal confession of faith. But what if we can't remember these historic details, what if we can't remember doing wrong and have no concept of sinfulness and repentance? What if we cannot recall whom we are required to believe in or have faith in? What sort of good news is it that requires us to take the initiative? What sort of Gospel is it that expects us to earn our salvation through acts of belief–for surely the word *'earn'* is appropriate if our salvation ultimately depends upon an act that *we* take.

But if God's gift and love extends to all, irrespective of their understanding or their memory; irrespective of their worthiness or their faithfulness–then we have quite a Gospel on our hands! But beware; it is a Gospel that offends all those who regard their own profession of faith as somehow being an integral part of that salvation story. It offends those who like to draw circles that allow some people to be on the inside and regard others as being on the outside. It offends those who feel that there are some people who have created a great gulf between themselves and God which will only be breached by some action on the part of the estranged . . . but what if that action has already been taken? What if one who has also been estranged, has stooped down to enfold the whole of humanity, and what if already the outcast and the marginalised, the confused and the bewildered, the healthy and the sick, the righteous and the unrighteous, the repentant and the unrepentant–what if they have all been received and welcomed, loved and forgiven by a gracious God who permits no barriers of ignorance, sinfulness or sickness to deflect his loving purposes. Now that would be good news! Now hear what I am saying, because that is not the dominant message coming from the majority of churches nor is it the view of most people who call themselves Christian as far as I can ascertain.

And isn't this precisely the challenge that dementia raises. For I firmly believe that each and every person with dementia is loved and accepted and enfolded by God; not because of *their* faithfulness but because of God's faithfulness.

And so after over forty years in the ordained ministry it has taken an engagement with dementia to reveal to me more surely than anything else has ever done that the good news that we have to share is that all are welcome, all are acceptable *and all are accepted*. This is the craziness of the Gospel, and it is good news–it is very good news for people with dementia, because wherever they might have been, they are on their way home and God will not forsake them, but will receive them, in fact already does receive them with a love that passes our understanding. We do well to remember that the experience of marginalisation and discrimination and the experience of helplessness and loneliness, of forsakenness and brokenness are at the very heart of the Christian revelation of God.

NOTES

1. T. Kitwood, *Dementia Reconsidered* (Buckingham: Open University Press, 1997).

2. R.S. Thomas, *Counterpoint* (Newcastle: Bloodaxe Books, 1990), 53.

3. R.S. Thomas, *RS Thomas: Autobiographies* (*The Absence* quoted in the Introduction) (London: Phoenix, 1998).

4. D. Keck, *Forgetting Whose We Are* (Nashville: Abingdon Press, 1996), 84.

5. Kitwood, *Dementia Reconsidered*, 46.

6. Psalm 22, Selected verses. *Book of Common Prayer* version.

7. D. Hammarskjold, *Markings* (London: Faber & Faber Ltd, 1964), 87.

8. J. Bayley, *Iris: A memoir of Iris Murdoch* (London: Duckworth, 1998).

9. L. Grant, *Remind me who I am again* (London: Granta Books, 1998).

10. G. Horst-Warhaft, "In the End is the Body" in *The Gospels in Our Image*, edited by D. Curzon (New York: Harcourt Brace & Co, 1995), 253.

11. Keck, *Forgetting Whose We Are*, 77.

12. J. Killick, *You are Words* (London: Hawker Publications Ltd, 1997), 42.

When Words Are No Longer Necessary: The Gift of Ritual

Malcolm Goldsmith, MSc, BSocSc

SUMMARY. This study is an exploration of non-verbal forms of communication which have become ritualised, particularly in the care of people with dementia. Rituals, which are culturally determined, may be inclusive or exclusive; they may lose their meaning or send out mixed messages, but in general they uphold the structure of society. There is a strong link between religion and ritual and for people with dementia, ritual may be extremely important in maintaining their sense of belonging within the community of faith. It looks at some of the issues to be addressed when worshipping with people with dementia. *[Article copies available for a fee from The Haworth Document Delivery Service: 1-800-342-9678. E-mail address: <getinfo@haworthpressinc.com> Website: <http://www.HaworthPress.com> © 2001 by The Haworth Press, Inc. All rights reserved.]*

KEYWORDS. Dementia, non-verbal communication, ritual/habit/symbol, worship

---

Malcolm Goldsmith is a priest in the Scottish Episcopal Church and Rector of St. Cuthbert's Church in Colinton, Edinburgh and is formerly a Research Fellow with the Dementia Services Development Centre in the University of Stirling.

Address correspondence to: Malcolm Goldsmith, 6 Westgarth Avenue, Colinton, Edinburgh EH13 0BD, Scotland (E-mail: Malcolm.Goldsmith@btinternet.com).

This paper was presented to the *Ageing, Spirituality and Pastoral Care in the 21st Century* conference in Canberra, Australia, January 2000 and subsequently amended for publication.

[Haworth co-indexing entry note]: "When Words Are No Longer Necessary: The Gift of Ritual." Goldsmith, Malcolm. Co-published simultaneously in *Journal of Religious Gerontology* (The Haworth Pastoral Press, an imprint of The Haworth Press, Inc.) Vol. 12, No. 3/4, 2001, pp. 139-150; and: *Aging, Spirituality and Pastoral Care: A Multi-National Perspective* (ed: Elizabeth MacKinlay, James W. Ellor, and Stephen Pickard) The Haworth Pastoral Press, an imprint of The Haworth Press, Inc., 2001, pp. 139-150. Single or multiple copies of this article are available for a fee from The Haworth Document Delivery Service [1-800-342-9678, 9:00 a.m. - 5:00 p.m. (EST). E-mail address: getinfo@haworthpressinc.com].

The role of ritual in the lives of people who are cognitively impaired, particularly in the area of dementia is an under-explored area and there is need for more research to be undertaken. There is much that can be learned from work done in the area of learning disabilities, particularly autism. What follows here are a number of observations that might encourage others to give time and thought to an important subject.

Each night I go through a ritual with my dog Slimmer. It has gradually evolved over the years until it has reached the point where it is an established part of both of our lives. No matter what has happened during the day, each night-time brings this little chain of events. The dog usually retires for the night before me; he seems to want to get to his 'box' at around 10pm and settle down, whilst I am usually an hour or two later. Before I retire, I reach up to take a dog biscuit from a box on a high shelf, and immediately the dog vacates his 'box' and has a good stretch. I move over, take out his special cushion, give it a good shake, and replace it in a more orderly way and the dog carefully treads over my arms and curls up in a ball. I then stroke him and offer him the biscuit. He always refuses two or three times and then, very gently, opens his mouth and lets me place the biscuit between his teeth—but first I have to run my fingers along them. Having done that, I give him a couple more strokes, wish him goodnight, switch off the light, close the door and go to bed! I have wondered how this little ceremony came about and what it means. I suppose it is a process of bonding—it is certainly a process of trust because he could have my fingers off in a moment. This is the same dog that barks ferociously at the postman, that races to and from without apparently paying the slightest heed to any instructions that I may be trying to give; a dog which for most of the time I would willingly give away to the first person who smiles at him. It is a dog with a mind of its own and yet, each night he needs this little ritual of care and trust.

This is an example of non-verbal communication and the ritual is, I suppose, our way of recognising that there exists between us a certain relationship which is somehow special. It reminds me of the time when my children were small and I would always call into their room to kiss them goodnight even though they were sound asleep and presumably were not aware of my presence (or were they?). Sometimes I regret that perhaps I take other important relationships too much for granted and I lack the means of expressing what they really mean to me. One of the commonest comments I hear at funerals is regret that people did not sufficiently express their love towards the deceased person when they were still with them.

In this chapter I want to begin to explore some of those non-verbal forms of communication which have, in some way or other become ritualised and see if there are ways in which we might harness them to create better patterns of care for people for whom communication by word is difficult. I have a special interest in working with people with dementia, but this area is also applicable to people with learning disabilities or to people who have had a stroke which may have affected their ability to speak or to communicate. Societies are held together largely by traditions and customs, ceremonies, habits and rituals. We all have routine patterns of behaviour, some of which may have become compulsive. We are surrounded by a host of symbols and concepts which come into play 'when words are no longer necessary'; some of these are religious and many of them are secular; some of them are individual and many of them are corporate.

It is salutary for Christians to remember that their Faith is a historical Faith and memory plays an important part in its transmission and practice and Protestantism in particular places a strong emphasis upon the intellect and the rational. The Word became flesh and dwelt amongst us, but ever since then we have been trying to turn that event and experience back into words, words and yet more words. Wonderful though words undoubtedly are, they are finite and often little more than mere approximations to the truths or emotions which we seek to convey by their use. T.S. Eliot wrote:

> Words strain,
> Crack and sometimes break, under the burden,
> Under the tension, slip, slide, perish,
> Decay with imprecision, will not stay in place,
> Will not stay still.[1]

(Printed with permission)

and it was my own Bishop and friend, Richard Holloway who wrote

> One of our greatest problems as humans is that our greatest gift, language, is also our greatest danger. We destroy ourselves by our words. The difficulty is that things are not what we say they are. The word 'water' is not itself drinkable. Words point to things, but they can never be the things they point to.

Speaking of the value of non-verbal communication and of imagery, he goes on to say:

> . . . it breaks through the frustration of language . . . art, particularly music and poetry, unites us with the thing beyond, places us in the midst rather than talks unceasingly and ineffectively about it . . . [2]

Just about every emotion can be expressed non-verbally: love, friendship, fear, jealousy, pleasure, anticipation, puzzlement, anger or hatred. We can see the power and effect of non-verbal communication in others and we are involved with it ourselves. It permeates every area of our life and becomes increasingly important when we are working or living with people who may have problems with language, be it foreign language, deafness or dementia.

Non-verbal communication can link us to our past as well as to our present, and it can provide us with hope for the future.

> . . . the infant explores the world through touch. The child cannot solve problems but learns by the repetition of actions reinforced by reward and punishment. Many of the early conditioned responses are learned at nonverbal level and seem to persist in advanced age, even in the presence of brain damage . . . due to the conditioning nature of early learning, nonverbal language takes on particular importance with confused patients in situations where words fail completely. Consequently, nonverbal communication, such as touch, may be successful when neural pathology prevents comprehension of verbal communication . . . unless repeated contact through touch is made with regressed patients, they will withdraw. And if there is an inability to speak, the isolation is even more profound.[3]

A Church of Scotland minister with Alzheimer's Disease was finding it more and more difficult to communicate by speech, but faithful and consistent visiting by a friend enabled them to find new ways of communicating. She described her visits to her minister friend in this way:

> The wilderness within you has been stripped
> only the graininess is left.
> Yet so much intact,
> despite the erosion of that sense of self;
> so much remaining
> which can cross the chasms
> when words get in the way of knowing

a touch, a smile–
with your engrained benevolence
you make me mindful of what humanness entails.
You have no cogent thought, and yet
your muddled words
are full of thoughtfulness.[4]

(Printed with permission)

One form of non-verbal communication is ritual, by which I mean a regularly performed procedure or a prescribed order of performing rites (when rites mean a body of customary observances characteristic of a church or a part of it, or an action or a procedure required to be done in a certain way).[5] Work done from a sociological perspective has developed our understanding of ritual. For followers of Durkheim there is a strong distinction made between the sacred and the profane and ritual is located clearly within the sacred area–"through rituals people correctly represent to themselves the pattern of relations in society." The Marxist approach see rituals as transmitting only false consciousness, mystifying people by misrepresenting the nature of social relationships.[6] For the majority of people, however, ritual is still understood as often repeated forms of behaviour, performed at appropriate times, which serve to bind societies (whether large or small) together and transmit values or meanings. In fact it has been argued that "the entire structure of society is upheld by rituals."[7] Rituals may contain words, but their essence is that the actions contain and communicate the inner meaning.

Much of the area covered by the word 'ritual' is also pertinent to our use of the word 'Habit.' Michael Young has pointed to four important functions of habit:

- They increase the skill with which we are able to perform certain actions
- They lessen fatigue because we no longer have to think through a process
- They not only economise on the amount of effort that is required for us to maintain ordinary, everyday routines; at the same time they release energy for those times when we need it, when confronted by something new, for instance, and so habits can become 'one of our chief tools for survival'
- They economise on the use of memory.[8]

In situations of dementia, care habit and ritual can become a gift when words are no longer necessary. Of course one might object that ritual is not always a gift and at times it can become a burden. Neurotic or obsessional behaviour is often ritualised–the compulsive washing of hands, the counting steps before crossing the road or other specific rigmaroles that must be adhered to before particular tasks can be done; though even these may be seen as positive ways of enabling the person to cope with the task in hand. As well there are the rituals which may be seen as gifts enabling us to communicate more effectively with people with dementia and there are also the rituals which some people with dementia begin to display which may themselves be attempts to communicate or which may be indications of a progressive neurological deterioration.

Sometimes it is the way that people behave that may be the first indication that there is such a problem:

> What we consider to be mental illness, Goffman argues, is the violation of the ceremonial rules of everyday life. Extreme and consistent violation of these rules is what gets one committed to a mental hospital in the first place. . . . the self depends on–one might also say, is created by,–the acceptable use of the ritual of ordinary social etiquette.[9]

Some rituals may lose their meaning and no longer meet a person's needs or they may be sending out mixed messages. In times of transition they may provoke considerable anxiety, cause embarrassment or give offence if we get them wrong. Take such simple examples as these customary forms of behaviour: do we stand up when someone enters a room or do men still 'touch their cap' when meeting a woman in the street? These may seem like little points of manners but they can assume great importance for someone with dementia.

These simple illustrations also serve as a reminder that rituals are culturally determined, age-related, gender-specific, influenced by place or affected by class. There is much ritual that is specific to the nation. Examples from Britain might be Remembrance Day, with the wearing of red poppies (the Peace Movement's white poppies caused quite a stir!); the Queen's broadcast on Christmas Day (how many families had rows on Christmas afternoon between those who wanted to watch and those who didn't!); Bonfire night on November 5th, remembering Guy Fawkes's attempt to blow up Parliament in 1605 (and thought by many to be the last honest man to enter Parliament!).

In addition there are family rituals as, for example, when you open your Christmas presents. Some families open them on Christmas Eve, others on Christmas morning and others in the afternoon. I was brought up as a child having presents in a pillowcase at the end of the bed–my wife wasn't, so when and how do the children get theirs? The ways in which people celebrate births, marriages and deaths also differ greatly. The processes are internalised and come out in ritualised behaviour, which is passed down through the generations. Language is often not necessary; people just *know* what they have to do. The person with dementia may not be able to remember or articulate details, but very often the cues will be sufficient for them to join in. But there may be problems for people in residential care if the staff are not aware of the family customs and practices, and if the cues are not picked up or are interpreted in different ways then the person with dementia may act in ways that other people deem to be inappropriate.

There is a great deal of ritual associated with religion. Much of it is conscious, in the ways in which worship is conducted, for example. That part is like the tip of an iceberg. A great deal of church ritual bypasses intellectual processes and is unconscious. It relates to some of our earliest encounters with religion and to practices encountered over the years that we may well have long since forgotten, but the impact that they made upon us remains deep within our psyche.

> The Catholic Church of yesterday had a texture to it, a feel: the smudge of ashes on your forehead on Ash Wednesday, the cool candle against your throat on St Blaise's Day, the waferlike sensation on your tongue in communion. It had a look; the oddly elegant sight of the silky vestments on the back of the Priest as he went about his mysterious rites facing the sanctuary wall in the parish church; the monstrance with its solar radial brilliance surrounding the stark white host of the tabernacle; the indelible impression of the blue-and-white Virgin and the shocking red of the Sacred Heart. It even had a smell, an odour, the pungent incense, the extinguished candles with their beeswax aroma floating ceiling ward and filling your nostrils, the smell of olive oil and sacramental balm. It had the taste of fish on Friday and unleavened bread and hot cross buns. It had the sound of unearthly Gregorian chant and flectamus genua and mournful Dies Irae. The church had a way of capturing all your senses, keeping your senses and being enthralled.[10]

Of course these are the things that poets write about or musicians and artists re-create in their own ways and we recognise the connection between our senses and the deepest levels of our being. When words are no longer necessary! This involvement of the senses is the context in which our rituals take place.

Take a rather different example, in this instance words were used but I could not understand them. Several years ago I attended a morning service in a remote part of Lesotho, in southern Africa. The service was in the local dialect. I could not speak or understand a word of it, and yet I could follow every part of the service because I understood the ritual of the Liturgy. It was interesting to note how, when I spoke at the service every word had to be translated for the congregation to understand, but when the priest celebrated the Eucharist I understood it all, though not a word was translated. My wife had a similar experience a few years ago when attending a Requiem Mass for a Polish neighbour in Edinburgh. The gift of ritual!

It is not therefore surprising that religious ritual can be extremely important when working with people with dementia because it can 'carry the person along.' They can relax in a group and maintain their presence in mainstream life without feeling over-anxious or causing too many anxieties for their carers. The person with mild to moderate dementia is still able to belong to the local congregation without standing out as being 'different' and they can continue in the worshipping life of the church without being required to engage in conversation. Of course it is important that churches are able to maintain the involvement of people with dementia even when their illness progresses much further, but by then it will require a conscious effort on the part of the congregation to maintain contact and to support and involve the person. In the earlier stages, people with dementia can be part of the community allowing the ritual of worship to speak for them. One person spoke to me about this experience saying it was like 'being carried along on a surfboard of love.'

Ritual can help a person to have meaning and self-identity. The Bar-mitzphah, the Military passing-out parade, the graduation ceremony at university are all ritualistic ceremonies which help provide a sense of identity which does not have to be spoken about. Rituals can link us into historic processes that are both reassuring and also affirming. 'This is the way that it is in our family; this is the way that we do things' and the person with dementia is as much a part of the family as anyone else and these rituals can help maintain their sense of belonging.

We need to be aware though that some rituals can also be *exclusive* as well as inclusive and can serve to marginalise and disempower people as well as affirming and empowering them. The Baptist at a High Mass may well feel utterly lost and bewildered by the ritualised processes, and a Roman Catholic at a Salvation Army meeting can feel equally uneasy and unsure of themselves. One of the effects of dementia, of course, may be to make the person feel increasingly unable to appreciate and recognise their own tradition. This was movingly described in Robert Davis' account of his 'journey into Alzheimer's Disease.'[11] The challenge to the carer is to discover just what are the experiences and rituals that affirm and which are the ones that do the opposite. Ritual is a gift when it empowers, but it can be a very heavy burden when it doesn't. It may be as easy to be trapped by ritual as it is to be liberated by it and some rituals seem to have the effect of shielding people from reality or preventing them from facing up to the possibilities of growth and empowerment.

A word about our use of symbols. Whilst rituals themselves may be symbolic (which is what possibly distinguishes them from habits), symbols also have their own specific function and it is one that can be useful in providing creative dementia care. The sensitive use of symbols can create an atmosphere of peace and acceptance, but in order to do this we need to identify the symbols that are meaningful to particular people.

Those responsible for providing worship may find it useful to draw up a checklist of symbols or symbolic actions that may or may not be helpful in their particular situation. This list is by no means exhaustive, but it can provide a starting point:

- Do we light candles? How many? Does it matter where they are placed?
- Do we use a cross (or crucifix)? Does it matter where it is placed?
- Do we use music? If we do, then what sort of music and is it live or taped'?
- Gregorian chant? Salvation Army band?
- Are we seeking to create a certain mood? Planning is of the essence here!
- Do we wear liturgical robes? Might this depend upon the age and background of those who will form the congregation?
- If ordained, do we wear a dog collar?
- A colleague of mine was advised against wearing his because a priest had once abused someone in his or her younger days–so how do we discover what is appropriate?
- Which version of the Bible do we use? Which hymns do we sing?

- These too are symbols of a truth to which they point, and we need to ensure that the symbolic element of the Word is not dimmed by our commitment to rational understanding.
- Is there an opportunity for physical contact?
- Sharing the peace? Holding hands? Giving an individual blessing to each person?

Eileen Shamy, who pioneered work in this area, reflected on worship in this way:

> I always wear my clerical collar, ecumenical alb, stole and cross and observe the colours of the liturgical year when leading worship for people with Alzheimer's Disease. Some ministers feel that they should not 'dress up' (their words) in the informal setting of the nursing home lounge. However, it needs to be understood that such memory cues are necessary to help many worshippers cue into 'church.' The nursing home lounge is now the only church space that the residents are likely to experience. I want to do everything possible to make it a holy place of Presence for them. That means clerical dress and vestments, flowers or candles, and a cross on the covered mobile feeding tray likely to be doing duty as an altar or communion table.
>
> More than this is required, of course–a good deal of praying long before, a conscious claiming of the company of the Holy Spirit and a complete dependence on the work of the Holy Trinity to build community, harmony and order.[12]

Being responsible for worship with people with dementia is a most onerous responsibility and it usually requires a great amount of preparation and also considerable time for reflection afterwards, as there is unlikely to be very much verbal feedback. We are dealing with situations where words are often not very helpful. The challenge is to find symbols and rituals that work instead. A colleague was recently holding a communion service in a dementia ward in a hospital and when it came to giving one patient the wafer he was met with a blank stare. Thinking quickly, he made the sign of the cross with the wafer and immediately the person opened their mouth and prayerfully received their communion.

A nursing home in Scotland, which specialises in dementia care, tried to address the problem of how to make Sunday a special day. For people in nursing homes each day can very often seem to be identical to the one that preceded it and tomorrow will seem to be the same as today. They aimed to ensure that each sensory aspect of the residents' experience was somehow different on Sundays. It began with breakfast, and Sunday was the day for bacon and the day gradually became associated with the smell and taste of bacon–and there is no smell quite like that of bacon! The visual impact to Sunday and one that could also be extended to touch was that the furniture was arranged and rearranged and the chairs in the Day Room were set out in a different way. Particular attention was paid to setting them out in a pleasant and relaxing way but also in a way that could easily be adapted for a service. Then there was special music and favourite hymns; hearing was recognised by ensuring that sounds that may have been identified with Sundays in the past were heard once again. None of these things in themselves was all that startling, but together they helped to ensure that Sunday had an altogether different feel to it. Ritual and symbol are a gift, when words are not really necessary.

> Bits of sentences collapse
> between brain and mouth:
> a computer file struck
> by a virus. Gaps which dangle
> between nouns are too big
> for leaps of inference;
> there is anxiety
> in both words and pauses;
> it is tempting to smooth
> their edges with inconsequentials.
> Having lost the past and future
> it seems that you are pure being;
> that you have made each instant
> your stillest dwelling.
>
> Yet you can smile that smile forever you
> to take us back, and lead us on;
> that simplest of complexities
> remains.[13]

(Printed with permission)

The smile, the gift–whether of ritual or not–when words are no longer necessary.

Perhaps this is one of the keys to creative dementia care, to be always on the lookout for gifts, for invariably, those who seek ultimately find.

NOTES

1. T.S. Eliot, *Four Quartets* (London: Burnt Norton V Faber and Faber 1944).

2. R.K. Holloway, *The Gospel according to Luke* (Edinburgh: Canongate Books, 1988), Introduction viii.

3. L. Seaman, "Affective Nursing Touch," in *Geriatric Nursing* (May/June 1982).

4. C. De Luca, in *Hearing the Voice of People with Dementia,* edited by MC Goldsmith (London: Jessica Kingsley, 1996), 24.

5. *Concise Oxford Dictionary* (1990 Edition).

6. *Concise Oxford Dictionary of Sociology,* edited by Gordon Marshall (1994).

7. R. Collins, "Erving Goffman on Ritual and Solidarity in Social Life," in *The Polity Reader in Social Theory* (Cambridge: Polity Press, 1994).

8. M. Young, "Time, Habit & Repetition in Day to day Life," in *Sociology: Introductory Readings,* edited by Anthony Giddens (Cambridge: Polity Press, 1997).

9. R. Collins, 1994.

10. V.J. Donovan. *The Church in the Midst of Creation* (London: SCM Press, 1989).

11. R. Davis, *My Journey into Alzheimer's Disease* (Amersham: Scripture Press, 1989).

12. E. Shamy, *More than Body, Brain and Breath* (Aotearoa, New Zealand: ColCom Press, 1997).

13. C. De Luca, 53.

The Spiritual Dimension of Caring: Applying a Model for Spiritual Tasks of Ageing

Elizabeth MacKinlay, RN, PhD

SUMMARY. This chapter describes a spiritual dimension of ageing using themes and a model for spiritual tasks of ageing, developed as a part of doctoral studies that examined spirituality amongst a group of independent-living older adults in Canberra and NSW. This model has been tested further and the model was confirmed through in-depth interviews of residents of nursing homes in the ACT. The first study identified six major spiritual themes from participant interviews. These were: ultimate meaning in life for each person, the way they responded to meaning, self-sufficiency versus despair, moving from provisional to final life meanings, relationship versus isolation in ageing and hope versus despair. *[Article copies available for a fee from The Haworth Document Delivery Service: 1-800-342-9678. E-mail address: <getinfo@haworthpressinc.com> Website: <http://www.HaworthPress.com> © 2001 by The Haworth Press, Inc. All rights reserved.]*

Rev. Dr. Elizabeth MacKinlay is Senior Lecturer at University of Canberra, Australia, Director of the Centre for Ageing and Pastoral Studies, at St. Mark's National Theological Centre, Canberra, and honorary assistant priest at the Anglican Church of the Good Shepherd, ACT.

The study *Spirituality in Older Residents of Nursing Homes* was supported by the Anglican Diocesan Foundation, Diocese of Canberra and Goulburn and Anglican Retirement Community Services (ARCS) Canberra and Goulburn.

[Haworth co-indexing entry note]: "The Spiritual Dimension of Caring: Applying a Model for Spiritual Tasks of Ageing." MacKinlay, Elizabeth. Co-published simultaneously in *Journal of Religious Gerontology* (The Haworth Pastoral Press, an imprint of The Haworth Press, Inc.) Vol. 12, No. 3/4, 2001, pp. 151-166; and: *Aging, Spirituality and Pastoral Care: A Multi-National Perspective* (ed: Elizabeth MacKinlay, James W. Ellor, and Stephen Pickard) The Haworth Pastoral Press, an imprint of The Haworth Press, Inc., 2001, pp. 151-166. Single or multiple copies of this article are available for a fee from The Haworth Document Delivery Service [1-800-342-9678, 9:00 a.m. - 5:00 p.m. (EST). E-mail address: getinfo@haworthpressinc.com].

151

KEYWORDS. Spirituality in ageing, meaning in life, vulnerability, transcendence, isolation, hope, wisdom, spiritual tasks of ageing

INTRODUCTION

Have you ever wondered why it is that some older people, while experiencing many disabilities and losses seem to have a wonderful sense of peace and joy in their lives, while others seem to exhibit a sense of despair? Anyone who has spent much time with older people will be able to point to examples of such people. Peace and joy versus despair. Real peace and joy flow from the depths of the individual human being, and are acknowledged as characteristics of the spiritual dimension. Further, it can be argued, peace and joy are signs of spiritual well being.[1]

So what is spirituality and how is it displayed in older adults? How can the spiritual dimension be mapped out to gain a greater understanding of what happens spiritually to people as they age? I want to suggest that it is helpful to look at spirituality in a developmental framework and that there are spiritual tasks of ageing. Further, I want to suggest that by looking at ageing from this viewpoint we may, first, more consciously develop our own spiritual dimension, and second, we may be more able to assist older people who may struggle to come to a sense of spiritual integrity in later life.

It is suggested that research is necessary to recover what are essentially naturally occurring skills of spiritual development in later life. These skills may need to be learnt by those who have lived in the 20th century. In fact the 20th century emphasis on science and technology may have been detrimental to many people who lacked the strategies required to develop the skills needed to grow spiritually. Yet, at the same time, that very research culture of the 20th century has made it possible to critically examine a human dimension that has until recently eluded study because the methods for its study were unavailable.

THE SPIRITUAL DIMENSION OF AGEING: A STUDY MAPPING SPIRITUALITY AND MEANING IN LIFE FOR A GROUP OF INDEPENDENTLY LIVING OLDER ADULTS

To begin, for me, it was necessary to learn more of what was happening to older people spiritually. There was plenty of anecdotal evidence, but it was important to go further and to attempt to increase the knowledge base to provide a more effective basis for practice. My doctoral studies mapped out the spiritual dimension of 24 independent-living older adults, of 65 years and older.[2] Further studies, following a similar process have focused on exploring the spiritual dimension of nursing home residents.[3]

The method used for the interviews was grounded theory.[4] Each person was interviewed at least twice, with a preliminary interview to establish relationship and collect demographic data and do an initial spiritual health inventory for elderly people (SHIE).[5]

The in-depth interviews in both studies used a broad framework of questions on meaning in life, growing older and God in their lives, for those who had a relationship with God. The questions allowed the participants to talk widely around the topic of meaning, seeking not to confine them to the researcher's interests. The samples of both studies included Christians and those who had no faith affiliation.

SPIRITUAL THEMES FROM THE STUDY
AND A MODEL OF SPIRITUAL TASKS OF AGEING

There were six major themes arising from the data collected from the doctoral study. Ultimate meaning, response to meaning, self-sufficiency versus vulnerability, wisdom and the search for final meanings, relationship versus isolation, and hope versus despair (see Figure 1).[6]

Theme: Ultimate Meaning for Each Person

The first theme arose naturally from the line of questioning on spirituality or ultimate meaning, in the life of each individual. Each person was asked: "Who or what gives greatest or deepest meaning to your life?" Most people were able to isolate this ultimate meaning to one or two components, for instance, relationship with others and for a number, with God and other people. Often this "other" was a spouse, if there was one. Some of the informants acknowledged multiple centres of meaning in their lives, such as finding meaning through music, art, and the environment. As could be expected from the demographic picture of ageing, those who were nursing home residents were less likely to have a spouse still living. On the whole members of this second group were both older and frailer. The nursing home participant average age was

FIGURE 1. Model of Spiritual Themes

Theme	Task
Ultimate meaning in life	to identify with what brings ultimate meaning
Response to meaning in life	to find appropriate ways to respond
Self-sufficiency/vulnerability	to transcend disabilities, loss
Wisdom/provisional to final meanings	to search for final meanings
Relationship/isolation	to find intimacy with God and/or others
Hope/fear	to find hope

78.7 years compared to the earlier study of independent-living older people of 75.3 years.

It is not surprising that there was a high level of response to the question of human meaning, because humans are characterised by their ability and propensity to attach meaning to objects and people in their lives. Meaning is open to review and change, at different points of the lifespan. Indeed, life without meaning leads to hopelessness.

Image of God

The material from in-depth interviews in this study allowed an exploration of each person's image of God, or sense of the other, as well as other aspects of spirituality. A life review of each person's spiritual and religious development was included in the interviews. It is contended that the image a person has of God (or gods), or indeed, the absence of such images, will play an important part in the whole of life experience for that individual.

Several questions were raised in the review of the literature: Does a person's image of God change across a lifespan? How might the God-image held by the person be related to hope? Or, in the absence of such images, what other factors might be relevant to the hope that an older person may claim in difficulties, such as suffering, loss, and/or facing death?

There were a number of images of God amongst the informants: a God of love, creator God, God of strength and power, a sense of God's presence. One informant who remarked, "God is there, but what in fact is it?" expressed this sense of a presence of God.[7] For some, there was a feeling of being distant from God. Indeed, a couple of people had constructed a god of their own and still others found meaning in life through a deep personal philosophy of life, without any concept of God. It is important to know what kind of image of God a person holds as this affects their sense of hope and well being; this is the centre from which people respond to life. A person who holds an image of a judgmental God will respond to life from that perspective, perhaps showing despair and hopelessness. On the other hand, a person who holds an image of a God of love will see hope even in the face of adversity.

Theme: Human Response to Ultimate Meaning

The second major theme was response to ultimate meaning. Subcategories of religious practice identified in human response to ultimate meaning from the in-depth interviews of independent-living older people were: worship, attending church, watching TV/listening to religious programs on radio, prayer, and reading Scripture. Some seniors practised meditation. Meditation was not understood by some of the participants. Some thought I was asking about medication rather than meditation, while some others recognised meditation only as an Eastern technique and seemed unaware of Christian meditation. Appreciation of music and art was an important mode for responding to meaning for some people. Some also spoke of the place of experience of "otherness" in their lives.

Frail elderly people and those with dementia may find it more difficult to respond to ultimate meaning as they would want, however, ritual can be an important way of connecting with these people. Amongst nursing home residents the need to worship seems to increase for at least some, who told me that they attend every service of any denomination that is conducted in the nursing home.[8]

A Model of Spiritual Tasks of Ageing

It seems from research in recent years that there is the potential for spiritual growth and development across the life span.[9] Using a developmental approach to spirituality in ageing, it is possible to identify tasks for each of the themes identified in the study of the spiritual dimension of ageing.[10] These tasks are to be accomplished in order to move to the wholeness that is the goal of human being. Drawing on the data from the doctoral study, a model of spiritual tasks of ageing was designed. Absolute wholeness is probably not possible in this life, but the goal is to continue growing in the spiritual dimension until death. The spiritual tasks become more urgent as people move closer to the end of life and begin to realise more clearly a sense of their own mortality.

The Spiritual Tasks of Ageing

These tasks arise from the themes identified from the data that relate to ultimate meaning for each individual. Each of the themes can be seen to have an associated task (Figure 2). The model developed from these themes and tasks is a dynamic one, with interaction between its components as indicated by the arrows (Figure 3).

Content of the Spiritual Tasks of Ageing

Content of the tasks will vary according to the individual's sense of ultimate meaning and their response to this. Thus for continued spiritual development it is necessary for the individual to become aware of and acknowledge their sense of ultimate meaning in life, and then to be able to respond to this in some way. That is, ultimate meaning and response to this meaning are a starting point for spiritual growth.

The model used in Figure 3 is a generic one and may be adapted to a variety of contents. For example, the model can be applied for an individual who is Christian, a member of other major faith groups, an agnostic, or an individual whose centres of meaning may be from a variety of other aspects, such as relationship, music and so forth.

Theme: Self-Sufficiency/Vulnerability
The Task: To Transcend Disabilities and Loss

> *Fear of increasing frailty: "I wouldn't like to be off my legs or lose my mind"*

This response from one of the informants was typical of responses from this group of older people. An important factor for all independent living older adults in my studies was perceived future vulnerability.[11] All acknowledged their apprehension as they pondered the possibilities of future dependence. There seemed to be a general consensus among those interviewed in-depth that older age came with dependency, loss of self-control and the possibility of mental deterioration. Some had already experienced the effects of physical disabilities and most lived with at least one chronic illness. However, the way they functioned in the face of disabilities varied a great deal.

FIGURE 2. Spiritual Themes and Tasks of Ageing: Each Theme Has an Associated Task

Spirituality in Ageing: Tasks

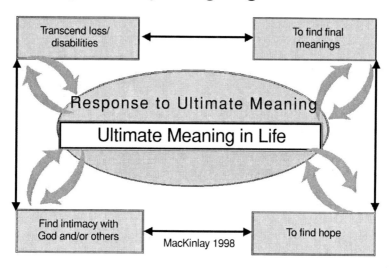

FIGURE 3. Generic Model of Spirituality in Ageing: Themes

Spirituality in Ageing: Themes

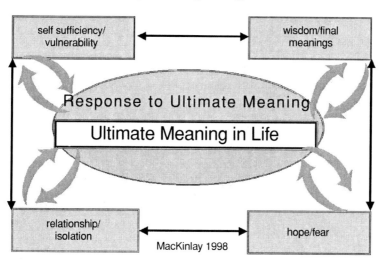

Various individuals expressed fears of the process of dying, but none expressed fear of death itself, even when asked directly. A number had had major surgery in recent years and/or live with chronic illness but still regarded themselves as being reasonably healthy. Fears expressed related to disabilities that would force life style changes on them, perhaps even amounting to the need for nursing home accommodation. Of particular concern to eight of the 24 who were interviewed is the possibility of developing Alzheimer's Disease. Two even spoke of losing control of their lives in this way as being a possible situation warranting suicide or euthanasia.

Betty remarked: "Oh, we're all afraid of dependence." She spoke of a friend who had Alzheimer's. Betty said she was fearful of becoming demented. Yet, also well known is the ability of many older people to transcend difficulties, such as loss, pain and suffering.

While fear of loss of control was an issue for the older independent-living group of informants, it was not an issue for most of those in nursing homes.[12] These nursing home residents had already experienced loss of control at first hand. Somehow, the reality did not seem to be as bad as the perception. These people were already frail, living with more than one chronic illness and vulnerable in a number of ways. Of this group, 45% expressed some fears, a much lower proportion than those living independently (100%). In fact, 55% said they had no fears at all. Yet the people in this study were much more frail and required assistance in several of the activities of daily living. They were in fact, experiencing the very things that those living in the community held as future fears.

Another question asked of the nursing home resident group was: "Is life still worth living?" to which 90% emphatically said, "Yes!" Even those experiencing many disabilities responded positively to this question. It seems so important to see life meaning from the view of the person whose life it is. All too often it is tempting to say, that the quality of life must be so poor for a particular individual that life may not be worth living. Often young nursing students have said to me: "I wouldn't ever want to be or live like that." Yet, time and again, these frail people affirm the importance of life to them. The perception of the individual older person must be taken into account when considering the value of life. Often, and to some extent understandably, health professionals value life from their own perspective, and fail to realise that the frail older person may be using a different frame of reference and values.

These people seem to have moved along a continuum from self-sufficiency towards vulnerability. These people had experienced vulnerability first hand and were at varying points of coming to terms with losses and disabilities. This process could be described as the development of self-transcendence. At the same time there are some older people who are weighed down by these same types of difficulties. Is it possible to assist these people to move to self-transcendence? This question was one that guided questions in this study.

Clements spoke of the stripping by society of the roles of earlier life.[13] Without spiritual resources, it may be found that when we lose mid-life roles there may be revealed a nakedness at the core of our being. A number of authors have written of the transition from doing to being that occurs in frail old age. This, perhaps obviously, was more evident amongst the nursing home residents than in those living independently. Tillich wrote of sanctification in ageing. All these are aspects of the process of transcendence.[14] The spiritual task of ageing is to transcend the disabilities and the losses, to move beyond the self.

The process of physical decline that is linked to the growth in spiritual development is loosely termed frailty. The term 'frailty' is poorly defined in the ageing literature, although the term is used frequently.[15] Most definitions of frailty agree that frail older adults are vulnerable and "have the highest risk of adverse health outcomes."[16]

Frailty is associated with underlying physiological changes of ageing that are evidenced by weakness, lowered energy levels, poor appetite, dehydration, and weight loss. This often leads to falls, injuries, increasing disability, dependency, being admitted to an aged care facility or hospital and death.

It is suggested that there may be an association between increasing frailty, an increased perception of approaching death and a move towards transcendence and the search for final meanings. Also importantly, a part of this phenomenon of increasing frailty is the move from doing to being. In a society that is so firmly tied to affirmation of people through their ability to contribute to society, this stage of being that occurs in the frailty of ageing may be confronting to family and carers. If those who care for frail elderly people understand the changes that are taking place in them, it is easier to provide appropriate care. Attitudes of ageism still exist in society and in some aspects of aged care. Valuing residents in nursing homes as "good residents" is at best unhelpful, at worst it is engaging in labelling and its effects can be demoralising and humiliating for residents, who may often sense these underlying attitudes. Those labelled as "good residents" may be ones who do not cause extra work for staff, for example, who can wait to be taken to the toilet, those who do not call out.

One woman who demonstrated transcendence over signs of physical decline was Carol, who lived alone. Carol said that she feared disease, falls, and intrusion into her life by others. A number of other issues were of concern to her as well:

> Because I have osteoporosis I'm inclined to have fractures of the spine, so I'm very limited in what I can do. I don't sit down and worry about it. It's if I wake up in the night, I imagine that I've got a growth, or I've got something wrong, and then I think about you know, what's going to happen to me and I worry a bit about whether there'll be the money to bury me.

Carol lived with a number of degenerative diseases, yet she had a good quality of life. She found that incontinence had made it too hard to continue studies at university, and this was a disappointment for her; however, she still lived a satisfying life in many other respects.

Of course there are considerable variations between individuals in the time of onset of physiological decline, and in fact a healthy life style can retard the decline; depending on the inherited potential for longevity. There are also considerable variations between individuals in the development of the psychosocial and spiritual dimensions. Interaction between the physiological, psychosocial and spiritual dimensions becomes more apparent in the later years, and while the physical body runs down, the psychosocial and spiritual dimensions continue to develop, unless blocked in some way.

THE MOVE FROM 'DOING' TO 'BEING' IN AGEING

In current Western societies identity is derived largely from what one's occupation is and when this is lost, particularly in frail older people, there is no longer an identity available for that person. When all other roles are stripped away, there remains a vulnerable human being. This seemed to be the basis for perceived future vulnerability for many of the informants in the study of well older people.[17] These people were experiencing the society of which they were a part. They were being conscious of the biological changes of ageing, the loss of roles, of work, of being mother, father, and the loss of loved ones. These people were beginning to feel the threat of finitude and anxiety common to all humans, described by Tillich.[18] The principle of sanctification referred to earlier in this chapter, in a context of vulnerability, is that of increasing transcendence, which is self-transcendence. Tillich stated that sanctification "is not possible without a continuous transcendence of oneself in the direction of the ultimate-in other words, without participation in the holy."[19] He said that while this is "usually described as the devotional life under the Spiritual Presence" it should not be exclusively used in this way. It may be that the individual might even restrict this aspect of their life; that prayer "may be subordinated to meditation, and religion in the narrower sense of the word, may be denied in the name of religion in the larger sense of the word." Even so, Tillich maintained " 'self-transcendence' is identical with the attitude of devotion toward that which is ultimate." [20]

This concept too is like Frankl's concept of self-forgetting, where the individual moves beyond the focus of self to focus on others.[21]

The process of moving from doing to being, it is suggested, is most probably a universal one; a process that becomes accentuated and more urgent in later life, as people realise that time is running out. While the term "sanctification" may not really be accessible to the general society, it is possible that the term "spiritual tasks of ageing" may be more acceptable both to older people and to the variety of carers who work with elderly people.

Theme: Wisdom/Provisional/Final Meanings
The Task: To Search for Final Meanings

Victor Frankl said that people attach provisional meanings to events in their lives, as these occur.[22] In the process of ageing, these meanings are re-examined in the light of further life experiences; growth and learning across the lifespan and eventually final, or ultimate meanings are constructed. It seems also that part of this move towards final meanings is connected with the development of wisdom in later life.

Mary, another woman living alone, had breast cancer about nine years ago. She only mentioned this in the context of being able to help and support others. She had a very positive attitude to life and health. This woman experienced many difficulties through her life, being divorced and bringing up a large family by herself, with few resources. Two of her adult sons were killed in separate accidents in recent years. She said: "I s'pose you get over it, you sort of get over it, but I mean it's always a sad spot, but then you think of all the other things you hear on TV, you know there's lots of people a lot worse off." She had always felt "kind of happy in myself." Although Mary never had a church background she developed a deep spirituality, she transcended difficulties in her life, and worked from a centre of internal regulation. She expressed a sense of joy through her painting and playing the violin. Wisdom was evident in her managing of her lifestyle, her ability to let go, and see a holistic perspective on life.

A definition of wisdom in ageing that recognises the spiritual dimension and used in this study is:

> An increased tolerance to uncertainty, a deepening search for meaning in life, including an awareness of the paradoxical and contradictory nature of reality; it involves transcendence of uncertainty and a move from external to internal regulation.[23]

Wisdom is acknowledged to be an important part of ageing, and part of this is a coming to final meanings. It is as Frankl has written, like the viewing of the many single frames from a movie.[24] It is only at the end of life that the whole movie can be run, and all the frames come together as a whole to make sense.

A spiritual task of later years is to go back over one's life and to review the single episodes of life, in context of the whole. Thus the task is editing, perhaps reframing past events and their provisional meanings; coming to a sense of final meanings in life. Here I am emphasising the spiritual aspect of reminiscence. It seems that for many people, this need only becomes evident as they perceive they are approaching the end of life and death. In our current society this task of reframing, of dealing with issues of life meaning, of guilt, of loss, of the need for forgiveness, and reconciliation with others and with God have become remote, perhaps even lost strategies. According to Heinz we have lost the ability to undertake the last career of life; that is, to die well.[25] Death has become medicalised and remote from families and friends. There is need to reclaim the whole of the life span, including the process of dying and relearn how to do this well, both as individuals and community.

Some of the frail older people in the nursing home study certainly demonstrated an increased tolerance to uncertainty, including an awareness of the paradoxical and contradictory nature of reality as outlined in the definition of wisdom used in these studies. This seemed to have developed out of necessity.

Theme: Relationship/Isolation
The Task: To Find Intimacy with God and/or Others

Relationship is an important aspect of being human. The human spirit longs for connection with others. For most, relationship with other people is vital; for some individuals relationship with God is all that is necessary; for others, it is both relationship with God and other people; for still others, the relationship is only with other people.

In ageing some who have shared intimately with another human being have lost that relationship through death. Along with the grief, it may be possible to develop new relationships; not replacing the loss, but relationships none-the-less, that will help fill the void left by death. In these cases new intimacy has to be developed, a difficult process for someone who has to begin again after so many years of being close to one particular person.

Older people who have no relationship with God also have a spiritual need for intimacy, and that need should be nourished in caring relationships with others. Only one older person in this study did not want a close relationship with other people. The spiritual task in ageing is to grow in intimacy with God and/or others. The spiritual journey, growing in intimacy with God, is likely to be a continuing one, although some older people do have conversion experiences and turn to God for the first time in later life. It is also noted that people who hold an image of a judgemental or punitive God may have difficulties in coming to a relationship of intimacy with God.

Theme: Hope/Fear/Despair
The Task: To Find Hope

A number of the informants in this study spoke of fears, particularly related to future perceived vulnerabilities, such as loss of control and possible suffering. For some people loss of loved ones and pain and suffering make it hard for them to maintain a sense of hope. The spiritual task is to find hope, perhaps even in the midst of loss and fear. Failure to thrive that is sometimes apparent in older adults may stem from a lack of hope. Tillich's model of sanctification seems to explain that move from despair to hope.[26]

In summary, the model of spiritual tasks was designed from the data of independent-living older people and tested with a sample of elderly nursing home residents. It seeks to explain the relationships between ultimate meaning and the ways that people respond to ultimate meaning. It outlines the move towards transcendence, the search for final meanings, the search for intimacy and for hope in later life. Although this model was designed from data from the interviews of older adults, it is not applicable only to older people, but in varying degrees at earlier points in the life-span. There is, perhaps, an increasing awareness of these spiritual tasks of ageing in the latter years of life.

APPLYING THE MODEL FOR SPIRITUAL TASKS OF AGEING

It is suggested that this model of spiritual tasks of ageing can be applied pastorally. An important starting point for practice is awareness of the spiritual needs of the individual. Ashbrook wrote that in care giving relationships we need to "risk being open to *their* perception of what is and what might be"[27] (my emphasis). Whatever the differences between older people, of the 75 who completed the spiritual health inventory, 92% said they had a faith.[28] This is important to note in planning chaplaincy and other pastoral services for older people. It is so important to reach out to the older person, to identify where they are spiritually. Are they in touch with their own inner needs? What kind of a belief system are they working from? It is important to identify, whether they have a deeply developed sense of the spiritual or whether they have no religious beliefs at all. Each person does have a spiritual dimension, and the challenge is for all who work with older people to be able to reach the older person at their point of need, that is, to connect with them.

HOW DO WE ASSIST OLDER PEOPLE WITH WORKING THROUGH THEIR SPIRITUAL TASKS OF AGEING?

The model of spiritual tasks of ageing may used to assess areas for spiritual need and growth.[29]

- Ultimate meanings: helping people to clarify their centres of meaning
- Response to meaning: assisting them to respond, by worship, music, art, reading, including use of Scripture. Affirming links with environment. Affirming their use of prayer. Identifying appropriate symbols of meaning
- Finding final meanings: journeying with them, assisting to reframe memories and experiences
- Transcending loss and difficulties: dealing with pain and suffering, assisting them in the grieving process, to move beyond and take up life again

- To establish intimacy with God and others: to find new intimate relationships. For example, with carers where there is no family; reconciliation with family may be important
- Finding hope: in attaining final meanings in life, reviewing and reframing past issues and looking to the future, for Christians, the ultimate hope of eternal life.

Settings for interventions and strategies may vary, from groups, including congregations for worship, small groups for spiritual reminiscence, groups for journeying spiritually, exploring art and music, and one-on-one sessions for spiritual life review therapy.

CONCLUSION

One of the most striking features of the older people interviewed in these two studies was the differences they showed in ageing. They had distinct and different personal histories, and brought skills based on these to meet their current needs and the demands made on them from the environment. Although there were broad aspects of experience that were common in a number of the spiritual journeys, the journeys of the informants were still definitely different.

The model developed in these studies gives a framework for interventions for health professionals, clergy and pastoral workers. This model may be applied to the many and varied spiritual needs of older people, acknowledging that individual older people will be at different places in their spiritual needs, and that these needs will be heightened at times of crisis for these older adults. Examination of the spiritual needs of older adults is leading to more effective ways of providing for quality of life in ageing. With increased application in practice of models of spiritual care in health and pastoral care, it is now possible to bring spiritual care into clear focus, as an important component of holistic care.

NOTES

1. Galations 5:22.
2. E.B. MacKinlay, "The Spiritual Dimension of Ageing: Meaning in Life, Response to Meaning and Well Being in Ageing" (doctoral thesis, LaTrobe University, 1998).
3. E.B. MacKinlay, "Study of Spirituality in Older Residents of Nursing Homes" (2000).

4. B.G. Glaser and A.L. Strauss, *The Discovery of Grounded Theory: Strategies for Qualitative Research* (Chicago: Aldine Atherton).

5. It is noted that the SHIE was not used with the nursing home group of people, as the results of SHIE from the doctoral studies were inconsistent with the material obtained from in-depth interviews. As well, factor analysis performed on the SHIE failed to support further use of this instrument.

6. MacKinlay, "The Spiritual Dimension of Ageing."

7. Response of one of informants in independent-living group.

8. This could be a time of social bonding for these residents.

9. J.W. Fowler, *Stages of Faith: The Psychology of Human Development and the Quest for Meaning* (San Francisco: Harper, 1981).

10. MacKinlay, "The Spiritual Dimension of Ageing."

11. Ibid.

12. Ibid.

13. WM. Clements, "Spiritual Development in the Fourth Quarter of Life," in *Spiritual Maturity in the Later Years,* edited by J.J. Seeber (New York: The Haworth Press, Inc., 1990).

14. P. Tillich, *Systematic Theology,* vol 3 (Chicago: The University of Chicago Press, 1963).

15. J.T. Stone, J.F. Wyman and S.A. Salsbury, *Clinical Gerontological Nursing: A Guide to Advanced Practice* (Philadelphia: W.B. Saunders Company, 1999), 315.

16. Ibid, 315.

17. MacKinlay, "The Spiritual Dimension of Ageing."

18. Tillich, "Systematic Theology."

19. Ibid, 235.

20. Ibid, 236.

21. V.E. Frankl, *Man's Search for Meaning* (New York: Washington Square Press, 1984).

22. Ibid.

23. Definition based on F. Blanchard-Fields, L. Norris, "The Development of Wisdom," in *Aging, Spirituality and Religion: A Handbook,* edited by M.A. Kimble, S.H. McFadden, J.W. Ellor, and J.J. Seeber (Minneapolis: Augsburg Fortress Press, 1995), 108.

24. Frankl, *Man's Search for Meaning.*

25. D. Heinz, "Finishing the Story: Aging, Spirituality and the Work of Culture," in *Journal of Religious Gerontology* 9 no. 1 (1994): 3-19.

26. Tillich, *Systematic Theology.*

27. J.B. Ashbrook, *Minding the Soul: Pastoral Counselling as Remembering* (Minneapolis: Fortress Press, 1996), 107.

28. MacKinlay, "The Spiritual Dimension of Ageing."

29. Ibid.

The Challenges and Opportunities of Faith Community (Parish) Nursing in an Aging Society

Antonia (Anne) M. van Loon, RN, PhD, MRCNA

SUMMARY. Faith Community Nursing is one form of health ministry that provides an opportunity to meet the challenges of an ageing society. This nursing is based on principles of communion, stewardship, service and transformation to promote the health of the community. Faith Community Nurses (FCNs) provide education, advocacy, counselling and assistance with care management to the faith community and beyond. Their work is complimented and supplemented by health ministry volunteers, using their knowledge and skills to build the social capital of the community. *[Article copies available for a fee from The Haworth Document Delivery Service: 1-800-342-9678. E-mail address: <getinfo@haworthpressinc.com> Website: <http://www.HaworthPress.com> © 2001 by The Haworth Press, Inc. All rights reserved.]*

KEYWORDS. Parish nursing, health ministry, pastoral care, social capital

Dr. Antonia (Anne) van Loon is a registered nurse, founding chairperson and current Director of Development of the 'Australian Faith Community Nurses Association' is a nurse researcher and academic at Flinders University, Adelaide, Australia.

Address correspondence to: Dr. Antonia van Loon, 5 Lowan Avenue, Glenalta, South Australia 5052 (E-mail: Antonia. VanLoon@flinders.edu.au).

[Haworth co-indexing entry note]: "The Challenges and Opportunities of Faith Community (Parish) Nursing in an Aging Society." van Loon, Antonia (Anne) M. Co-published simultaneously in *Journal of Religious Gerontology* (The Haworth Pastoral Press, an imprint of The Haworth Press, Inc.) Vol. 12, No. 3/4, 2001, pp. 167-180; and: *Aging, Spirituality and Pastoral Care: A Multi-National Perspective* (ed: Elizabeth MacKinlay, James W. Ellor, and Stephen Pickard) The Haworth Pastoral Press, an imprint of The Haworth Press, Inc., 2001, pp. 167-180. Single or multiple copies of this article are available for a fee from The Haworth Document Delivery Service [1-800-342-9678, 9:00 a.m. - 5:00 p.m. (EST). E-mail address: getinfo@haworthpressinc.com].

167

INTRODUCTION

Ageing provides a variety of physiological and social changes that invariably impact on health. It is these changes that Faith Community Nursing (also known as Parish Nursing or Pastoral Nursing) is potentially able to address. Faith community nursing is a specialist nursing practice distinguished by its endorsement of a faith-based perspective of the person, which focuses nursing care on integration, nurture and restoration of the whole person in all their dimensions (physical, intellectual, psychosocial, spiritual). Faith community nurses (FCNs) help people with existing diseases or complex conditions to better manage their illness, thus enabling them to maximise their quality of living. However, FCNs primarily focus on promoting the preconditions for personal and community health, by fostering healthy relationships, addressing social justice issues and providing education and support to people regarding faith and health issues. All these activities are undertaken in the context, and with the support of the faith community. The FCN's clients are not restricted to the faith community; thus the program has the capacity to reach into the wider geographic and/or cultural community that group serves.[1]

THE CHALLENGES AND OPPORTUNITIES

Loneliness and Isolation

Increasing numbers of older persons will face their senior years alone. Currently two thirds of Australians (65-75 years) are married, but this figure is set to change radically in the future. Fewer people are choosing to marry, family sizes are decreasing, divorce and separation rates are increasing, so many people are left without the support of partners or children in their senior years.[2] The increasing mobility of Australian society has contributed to these changing family dynamics, with many children living far away from their aging parents. This fragmentation of marriages and families takes an emotional toll on relationships between children and their parents, leaving many elderly disconnected and isolated from family.

Literature produced during the International Year of Older Persons (1999) by the Body Shop[3] included a broad sheet of comments responding to the statement 'In my life ageing means to me . . .' The responses ranged from ambivalence to rage, with some deeply personal accounts of loss and grief associated with losing youth, status, and loved ones. Several people commented on the intense loneliness they experienced when they were unable to get around like they used to. This loneliness was often accompanied by feelings of hopelessness, uselessness, and boredom. These are core spiritual issues that faith communities can and should address.

One method of addressing isolation and loneliness is to create support networks that connect people and nurture relationships. Health is affected and effected by relationships; thus ministering to older Australians must be focused on improving the quality of relationships within the faith community. Nurturing spirituality involves creating, sustaining and restoring relationships within the dimensions of the individual (body, mind, spirit); between the person and other people (family, significant others, and community–both local and global); between the person and the created environment; between the person and God.[4] These four relational areas impact on individual and community health and wellbeing, because positive relationships are a significant hallmark of community health. A recent study undertaken in South Australia's western suburbs by Baum[5] clearly demonstrated that 'social participation relates to health status independent of socio-economic status and age.' There is no organisation in Australian society other than the faith community, which regularly and voluntarily congregates people of all ages and facilitates the development of long-term relationships across the life span. It brings people of diverse backgrounds and ages together into meaningful relationships where they have the freedom to bless each other, and be blessed, to share and have a share, to partake and give, to forgive and be forgiven. People may mistakenly think relationships need to be perfect to be of benefit, but in a community people learn from each other's victories and mistakes. Relationships can grow in the midst of trial and testing. The key to growth lies in the connection and common grounding in love for God, enabling people to transcend differences, forgive and love again. This makes the faith community a fertile ground for the development of social capital, which no government can simulate, yet its powerful impact on health is often taken-for-granted by the church, the society and governments! The challenge the faith community faces in this new century is connecting people into loving relationships, limiting human isolation, and maximising communion.

Challenging the Stereotypes of Older Persons

Faith communities must challenge negative stereotyping and subsequent silencing of the older person's voice. Children are asked, 'What would you like to do when you grow up?' Teenagers may be questioned 'What would you like to do after you finish high school?' Adults are queried, 'What sort of work do you do?' Retirees are requested, 'What are you going to do with your time now you have retired?' What is the 80-year-old asked? Older people are being invited less to express opinions about issues affecting them, and this society. I have heard the comment from several older people that they feel as if society considers them 'well past their use-by-date.' Faith communities must challenge the silencing of older voices, and stop perpetuating the negative stereotypes associated with aging. Age does not alter God's intention for his people.[6] Age is no barrier to spiritual growth and service in the faith community. All voices are part of the body and worth listening to. All ages have a positive life affirming contribution to offer, and be valued for.

These stereotypes can be challenged by inviting people to share their story and demonstrate how 'my story' and 'their story' fit into 'His (God's) story.' This can be done by activities such as sharing in small groups, interviews (live, or in the church bulletin), children's talks, buddy systems, pastoral partnerships and special evenings.

Older members can contribute a sense of balance about life, where a living hope born from a nurtured spirit replaces the often-transient desires on which younger generations focus. Many older persons look back on life seeing clearly their losses and mistakes. They can share how they found meaning in life and how they continue to fulfil their purpose in life.

Sharing personal stories is a worthwhile community building experience. One memorable evening I organised for our youth program older members sharing their experiences during World War II with the youth. The stories of faith in the midst of adversity had a profound impact on all present. It was a cathartic experience for many older people with tears flowing freely, and it created a new depth of understanding in our community between the generations.

Getting the Church to Rediscover the Value of 'Community'

Some churches need to rediscover the value in communing with each other and God, learning how to become a faith community, rather than being a weekly meeting place. Crabb[7] elaborates:

Because we have become a nation of individuals-with-problems, we have missed our destiny to be people-in-community. We go to impersonal churches where programs outnumber relationships, and we schedule appointments with personal experts who sell an hour of relationship per week.

The Biblical analogy of a shepherding illustrates how the shepherd brings sheep into God's pastures to receive nourishing. God, as shepherd, provides all that people need, but God's people, as under-shepherds, must direct people into God's 'pastures.' The Church as under-shepherds must recover isolated individuals and return them to the community where encouragement, nurture and protection are available. A key part of the church's existence is to provide support, safe-keeping and sustenance for all people.

The faith community can provide people to listen, accompany, and love in simple ways such as bringing older persons to activities, transporting them to worship services, or alternatively ensuring they receive regular visitors when they can no longer make the journey to worship. In this way they experience a sense of connection to the faith community. The pastoral care and health ministry of the faith community provides support for older people in the congregation. It mobilises the resources of the congregation to supplement and compliment those already available in the community through the health and social welfare systems. Once the needs within the faith community are met the focus broadens to include people in the wider community. The creation of pastoral partnerships is one key aspect of the health ministry program. It makes each person responsible for one to three other people, thus ensuring all the group are cared for.[8] The entire faith community has the opportunity to support this health ministry, by using their particular gifts, talents, professional expertise and networks of contacts.

THE BIBLICAL PRINCIPLES
BEHIND FAITH COMMUNITY NURSING

The Australian faith community nursing model was developed in Christian churches and is based on the following Biblical principles:

The Principle of 'Stewardship'

A steward is one who manages a household, or is entrusted with something valuable and acts as its guardian or curator.[9] In the New Testament a good steward had qualities of forgiveness, reconciliation, liberation, accountability, investment, giving, compassion and mercy. Stewardship then describes how one accepts and carries out their delegated responsibility. For the faith community stewardship involves utilising the unique gifts and talents of all members in service to others. God calls people to care for creation as 'good stewards' obligating Christians to address environmental issues impacting on health such as disposable goods, pollution and land fill, but also to care for the earth's people and for ourselves. This implies guardianship over the poor and disenfranchised people groups locally and globally, such as sufferers of HIV, alcoholics, the homeless, the mentally ill, the abused, those with memory disorders and more.

The Principle of 'Communion'

The Bible illustrates the importance of communion with God and with each other through Holy Communion (Eucharist, or Lord's Supper). One may enter the community as a solitary individual but through communion *"With them, I belong to Christ. To them, through Christ, I belong. To me, through Christ, they belong. No longer am I isolated from them. We share life. We share Christ."*[10] Communion is the basis for the gathering of people that make up the Christian faith community. Communion involves sharing and having a share, partaking and participating. Communion is only built in the 'we,' not the 'I,' or the 'us.' It is based on *'being' with another, not just 'doing'* for another--sharing their suffering, touching their hurts, being silent with them in their despair, and staying with them. Communion involves hearing, listening, talking and appropriate touching. Creating community involves building and fostering patterns of relating, breaking down barriers through sharing, giving, receiving and being. This is the principle behind the health promoting capacity of life lived in a caring Christian faith community.

The Principle of 'Servanthood'

A servant is an active agent, always accountable and under authority, for the Christian that is God's authority.[11] It is someone who has chosen to use their talents, rather than been coerced. A servant is a friend, confidant and partner of all, not just those whom one might select to include into their circle of friends.[12] A servant is not a slave, or a doormat, rather a servant lives daily to reflect and represent Christ in the world. A servant looks for and fills the gaps wherever he/she is, and in this way will always be unconsciously involved in the world's needs. Servanthood is focused on attitude rather than action, our nature rather than our lifestyle. Observing other role models in our community, where the best leaders are often also the best servants, learns the art of serving. Finally, a servant measures success in faithfulness to God's calling, a point worth pondering in this outcomes and performance based society!

The Principle of 'Transformation' → 'Reconciliation' → 'Restoration'

The overarching goal of all FCN functions is transformation that leads to reconciliation and restoration in all dimensions of the person.[13] This includes transforming the individual's and the community's conceptualisation of health and healing, empowering people to act in ways that enable them to respond positively to life and improve their well-being. The transformative process is a dynamic, life-long journey that enables us to grow closer to Christ and become more like him in every dimension of our lives. Thus all FCN functions aim to nurture spiritual growth and clarify the relationships between faith and health.[14]

The act of living requires responses to changes, stressors and perceived stressors that may originate within or external to the person. Stressors can range from tangible microbes to mystical spiritual issues. All individuals must adapt to stressors, remove them, ameliorate their effect, or build up inner resources to prevent stressor impact. Certain life changes are in our control, such as some relational and lifestyle issues, but other stressors are outside the person's control, such as developmental changes and environmental crises. The whole person must respond by finding new ways to live and be in the world. The FCN can assist the person to respond to their changing conditions by developing new and alternative patterns of living.

FCNs promote health by facilitating the transformative growth that enables a person to respond positively to change. Peterson notes successful health ministries are built on transformation within the faith community regarding 'reconceptualisation of the meaning of health, and empowering people to act in ways that improve their well-being.'[15] He adds the biomedical interpretation of health that currently exists in the faith community is similar to the rest of society, who respond to illness by handing over self-care to a professional, and respond to wellness by ignoring it, making little effort to maintain it. Thus much FCN work focuses on creating and fostering positive relationships as the foundation for the personal growth and transformation that nurtures health.

The final goal of the transformative process is restoration. This process involves re-establishing relationships, bringing about reconciliation between people and God, and reconstructing lives after loss experiences. FCNs help people restore relationships disrupted by sickness, separation, divorce, death and so on. Much effort is directed to providing counselling, resources, advocacy and mediation to achieve restoration, aiming to help people through crisis and loss events in their life, to re-establish and reconcile relationships when possible, or ameliorate stressor impact if restoration is not an option. The FCN may be a source of comfort and reassurance in times of distress; however, people in significant distress and dysfunction are referred to skilled counsellors, pastors and specialist health professionals. Reconciliation with God can and does occur (often without intentional effort) by compassionate presence in times of distress, simply being with the person in their despair. When restoration and reconciliation are not an option, the FCN aims to help clients reconstruct their life by adjusting to changed situations.

The FCN model of health ministry is based on these four principles, which are then translated into practice to include six key FCN functions.

THE KEY FAITH COMMUNITY NURSING FUNCTIONS

The key functions of the faith community nurse role may be summarised using the acronym 'HEALTH.'[16]

Helping with Resource and Referral

The FCN liaises between the individual and the faith community, and the individual and other health and community services. The FCN is able to negotiate, access and assist entry into health services and local community support networks of which people may be unaware. This resource and referral activity occurs within the faith community and beyond. The aim is to better manage and coordinate care for individuals and communities.

Education and Facilitation

The FCN uses various methods to educate individuals and facilitate small groups in the community in the areas of: lifestyle factors, faith and relationships, health enhancement activities, illness risk reduction, disease management, environment awareness, social justice issues and other health and well-being issues that are pertinent to the group of people the FCN serves.

Advocacy and Mediation

FCNs are called upon to publicly support, uphold, recommend or defend a particular position/person. This involves interpreting points of view and helping people to 'see' another perspective. Thus this function can include mediation to bring about agreement and/or reconciliation between people. This function includes prayer with and for clients and their families.

Listening and Counseling

Personal and small group counselling and advocacy is an important aspect of the role: helping people with health problems, listening and advising as required, supporting and recommending referral if required, in addition to home visits and monitoring progress. The role includes offering knowledge of viable options to assist the individual to make informed choices in a supported environment.

Training and Coordinating Volunteers

The FCN coordinates, educates, trains and supports groups of ancillary workers and volunteers who sustain the health ministry within the faith community.

Helping with Care Management

The FCN may assist clients with existing illnesses, complex conditions and/or disabilities to manage their condition aiming to prevent exacerbations and/or limit complications. The FCN's holistic approach to care management considers the client, their family, the client environment and the faith community, when developing care management with the client.

Since the development of the FCN role in Australia, I am frequently asked why the professional of choice for health ministry should be a nurse. It is therefore useful to briefly discuss these issues in the context of this paper's proposal to use an FCN program to meet the challenges and opportunities of an aging society.

Why Should a Nurse Conduct This Health Ministry?

Health ministry does not require a nurse; rather it needs a team approach. However, there are distinct advantages to having a nurse as the key organising professional. These are summarised by Westberg when he claims, 'The nurse has the sensitivity–the peripheral vision, I call it to see beyond the patient's problems and verbal statements. She can hear things left unsaid. And she is the best listener.'[17] Westberg asserted nurses have the requisite scientific expertise, special gifts in caring, and excellent people skills required for effective health ministry. He notes nurses command respect from the community, and are trusted by people, enabling them to open up to a nurse. Interestingly nurses in Australia consistently poll number one, as the most ethical profession, exceeding the medical profession and ministers of religion.[18] Westberg goes on to note that nurses use their 'peripheral vision' to identify people who they know need to be visited quickly, thus he states nurses are the profession of choice for faith community based health ministry.[19] I would add that nurses have a broad knowledge that crosses many discipline boundaries, making them an ideal 'navigator' of an increasingly complex health system, and an excellent resource person to the faith community.

It is worth noting that nursing has its historical roots in the early Christian church, in the deaconess role of caring for the sick, widowed and orphaned (see Romans 16:1-2 NIV). From these beginnings developed the religious orders of sisters and brothers who continued caring for the sick and travelling pilgrims, in hospitals and homes throughout history. The deaconess role was revitalised by Pastor Theodore Fliedner in Germany in the 18th century. Inspired by the work of Dutch deaconesses and British prison reformers such as Elizabeth Fry, Fliedner began a hospital and deaconess training institute in Kaiserwerth in 1836.[20] Fliedner realized the need for women to work to avoid the hunger and poverty that was leading many into criminal activity and subsequent imprisonment. The deaconesses were provided an income and the society received their charitable works amongst the poor, sick, orphans, and other women in prison. Kaiserwerth nurses were educated in nursing theory, clinical care, ethics and religious doctrine. By the late 1850s, nurses trained at Kaiserwerth were in fifty-nine foreign stations throughout America, Asia, and Europe.[21] Florence Nightingale was one of many nurses trained at Kaiserwerth, who changed the face of nineteenth century nursing to reclaim care of the whole person: body, mind and spirit.

The current 'parish nurse' role has revamped the deaconess role. It was commenced in the United States of America (USA) in 1984 by a Lutheran pastor, the late Reverend Granger Westberg.[22] He was an advocate of holistic health centres that he helped to trial in the 1970s.[23] These centres used a medical doctor, social worker, pastor and a nurse to provide care. They were costly and unable to be sustained once initial university and foundation monies ceased. Westberg identified that the 'glue' which held the teams together were the nurses.[24] Nurses had knowledge across disciplines and provided the professional linkages for quality care. Westberg commenced a trial in 1984, which placed six nurses in six churches in the Chicago area.[25] Suffice to say, the trial was a success and parish nursing has flourished in the USA. There are now approximately 2,000 nurses who have undertaken the basic preparatory course endorsed by the International Parish Nurse Resource Centre, and there are estimates of around 4-6,000 parish nurses across the USA.[26] Faith community nursing has also commenced in Canada, Korea, New Zealand and Australia.

Faith community nursing formally commenced in Australia in 1996 when several faith community nurse ministries commenced in South Australia, in a demonstration project initiated by doctoral candidate Anne van Loon. There is word of nurses having occasionally held pastoral positions in Australian churches some years prior to the formal commencement of this project, but its recognition as a nursing specialty has occurred since the commencement of the 1996 demonstration project. Five Christian faith communities (1 Anglican, 2 Roman Catholic, 1 Lutheran and 1 ecumenical Christian agency working with homeless youth) developed the role to meet the existing needs and mission of their own faith community. The data was collected over 1997/1998 and a model for practice developed from this data.[27] The concept of health ministry is growing as faith communities see the potential afforded by faith community nursing. The Australian Faith Community Nurses Association (AFCNA) was formed in 1996, and has a mandate to provide FCNs with support, education, resources and networking opportunities, whilst engaging in promotion and professional lobbying regarding faith community nursing (AFCNA 1999).[28] Faith community nursing has been developed in Australia with the specific aim of providing the faith community with a structured ministry focus to meet the health needs of a changing society, which includes an aging society.

CONCLUSION

The twenty-first century holds many challenges with an ageing population who are experiencing increased loneliness and isolation and many western countries experiencing difficulties meeting the needs of the frail and dislocated elderly. Negative attitudes regarding older people are sowing the seeds of an 'ageist' society. It is easy to feel hopeless and powerless about the future, but these challenges may be viewed as opportunities for the faith community to reassert its capacity as a healing community.

The Christian Church has been called to follow Jesus' lead, and go out to love and serve each other, and the people of the world. The health ministry of the faith community nurse is a response to this call. FCNs provide whole person care (body, mind and spirit) while nurturing the growth towards wholeness in and through Christ. An ageing society needs the faith community to respond with a positive and appropriate response to their changing needs and seize the opportunities before it.

NOTES

1. A.M. Van Loon,"Creating a conceptual model of Faith Community Nursing in Australia using Participatory Action Research" (Unpublished doctoral dissertation, Flinders University, Adelaide, South Australia, 1999).

2. P. Hughes, "Ministry in the year of older persons" in *Pointers* 9 no. 4 (December 1999): 1-5.

3. IYOP 1999, "The Body Shop Partnership," in *Update Coalition '99 South Australia* 6(2) (November/December 1999): 6.

4. Van Loon, "Creating a conceptual model of Faith Community Nursing."

5. F. Baum, "Being social is good for your health" in *Research Matters* 8 no. 4 (December 1999): 1.

6. Psalm 92:12-15.

7. L. Crabb and D. Allender, *Hope When You Are Hurting* (Michigan: Zondervan, 1996), 183.

8. 1 Peter 5:3.

9. R. Christopher, "Stewardship in nursing," in *Concepts in Nursing: A Christian Perspective,* edited by R. Stoll (Madison, USA: InterVarsity Christian Fellowship USA, 1990).

10. J. Wessman, "Community building: A Process in Christ centred nursing care," in ibid., 191.

11. Hebrews 13:17.

12. E.M. Fordyce, "Servanthood: Service through nursing," in *Concepts in Nursing: A Christian Perspective,* edited by R. Stoll (Madison: InterVarsity Christian Fellowship USA, 1990), 91.

13. Van Loon, "Creating a conceptual model of Faith Community Nursing."

14. Ibid.

15. B. Peterson, "Renewing the church's health ministries: Reflections on ten years' experience," in *Beginning a Health Ministry: A 'How to' Manual,* edited by M. Arenas and J. Goodnight (California: Health Ministries Association, 1994): 2-11-19.

16. Van Loon, "Creating a conceptual model of Faith Community Nursing."

17. G.E. Westberg, "Parish nursing's pioneer," in *Urban Health* (October 1989): 2.

18. See *The Australian*, 21/5/1998.

19. G.E.Westberg, "A historical perspective: Wholistic health and the parish nurse," in *Parish Nursing: The Developing Practice*, edited by P.A. Solari-Twadell, A.M. Djupe and M.A. McDermott (Park Ridge, USA: Lutheran General Health System, 1990b).

20. M.P. Donahue, *Nursing the Finest Art: An Illustrated History* (St Louis, USA: Mosby, 1985), 235.

21. J.E. Olson, *One Ministry, Many Roles: Deacons and Deaconesses Throughout the Centuries* (St Louis, USA: Concordia, 1992).

22. G.E. Westberg and J. Westberg McNamara, *The Parish Nurse: Providing a Minister of Health for your Congregation* (Minneapolis, USA: Augsburg Press, 1990a).

23. D.A. Tubesing, *An Idea in Evolution: History of the Wholistic Health Centers Project 1970-1976* (Illinois, USA: Wholistic Health Centers, 1976).

24. Westberg, "A historical perspective: Wholistic health and the parish nurse," 27.

25. G.E. Westberg, "Churches are joining the health care team" in *Urban Health* (October 1984).

26. P.A. Solari-Twadell & M.A. McDermott, eds. *Parish Nursing: Promoting Whole Person Health Within Faith Communities* (Thousand Oaks, USA: Sage Publications, 1999).

27. Van Loon, "Creating a conceptual model of Faith Community Nursing."

28. AFCNA, Australian Faith Community Nurses Association, *Faith Community Nursing: A Resource Manual* (Adelaide: Australian Faith Community Nurses Association, 1999).

REFERENCES

ABS, Australian Bureau of Statistics. *Census of Population and Housing, 1911-199*, Canberra, Australia: Australian Government Publishing Services, 1996.

AFCNA, Australian Faith Community Nurses Association. *Faith Community Nursing: A Resource Manual.* Adelaide, South Australia: Australian Faith Community Nurses Association, 1999.

Australian Nurses our most ethical profession, *The Australian* 21/5/1998 (June 21, 1998): 12.

Baum, F. "Being social is good for your health." *Research Matters* 8(4) (December 1999): 1-3.

Christopher, R. "Stewardship in nursing." In *Concepts in Nursing: A Chrisitian Perspective*, edited by R. Stoll. Madison, USA: InterVaristy Christian Fellowship USA, 1990.

Crabb, L. and Allender, D. *Hope When You Are Hurting.* Michigan: Zondervan, 1996.

Donahue, M.P. *Nursing the Finest Art: An Illustrated History.* St Louis, USA: Mosby,1985.

Droege, T.A. "Premises and promises of health and healing." In *That It May Be Well With You* edited by R. Hardel and J. Mull. Minneapolis: Augsburg Youth and Family Institute, 1994.

Fordyce, E.M. "Servanthood: Service through nursing." In *Concepts in Nursing: A Christian Perspective*, edited by R. Stoll. Madison, USA: InterVaristy Christian Fellowship USA, 1990.

Hughes, P. "Ministry in the year of older persons." *Pointers* 9(4), (December 1999): 1-5.

IYOP (1999). "The Body Shop Partnership." *Update Coalition '99 South Australia* 6(2), (November/December 1999): 6.

NIV *The Holy Bible: New International Version*. International Bible Society. Colorado, USA: Zondervan Bible Publishers, 1988.

Olson, J.E. *One Ministry, Many Roles: Deacons and Deaconesses Throughout the Centuries*. St Louis, USA: Concordia, 1992.

Peterson, B. "Renewing the church's health ministries: Reflections on ten years' experience." In *Beginning a Health Ministry: A 'How To' Manual*, edited by M. Arenas and J. Goodnight. California, USA: Health Ministries Association, 1994: 2-11-19.

Solari-Twadell, P.A. and McDermott, M.A. eds. *Parish Nursing: Promoting Whole Person Health Within Faith Communities*. Thousand Oaks, USA: Sage Publications, 1999.

Tubesing, D.A. *An Idea in Evolution: History of the Wholistic Health Centers Project 1970-1976*. Illinois, USA: Wholistic Health Centers, 1976.

Van Loon, A.M. "Creating a conceptual model of Faith Community Nursing in Australia using Participatory Action Research." Unpublished doctoral dissertation, Flinders University, Adelaide, 1999.

Westberg, G.E. "Churches are joining the health care team." *Urban Health* (October 1984): 34-36.

Westberg, G.E. "Parish nursing's pioneer." *The Journal of Christian Nursing* 6(1) (Winter 1989): 26-29.

Westberg, G.E. and Westberg McNamara, J. (1990a). *The Parish Nurse: Providing a Minister of Health for Your Congregation*, Minneapolis, USA: Augsburg Press.

Westberg, G.E. (1990b). A historical perspective: Wholistic health and the parish nurse, In Solari-Twadell, P.A., Djupe, A.M, & McDermott, M. A. (Eds.) *Parish Nursing: The Developing Practice*, Park Ridge, USA: Lutheran General Health System.

Wessman, J. Community building A process in Christ centred nursing care, In Stoll, R. (Ed) *Concepts in Nursing: A Chrisitian Perspective*, Madison, WI, USA: InterVaristy Christian Fellowship USA. 1990.

EPILOGUE

Radical Discipleship
for an Ageing Society

Stephen Pickard, PhD

*Homily preached on the Feast of St. Paul, 22 January 2000
Chapel of John 23, Australian National University*

Conference on Ageing, Spirituality and Pastoral Care
for the Twenty-First Century
Canberra, Australia

"The time is short." Who says so? In the first instance the prophet of
is none other than the Apostle Paul, whose feast day we celebrate today.
He writes with a sense of urgency as if time were running out: "The time
is short." Paul has been gripped by a reality far more exciting, urgent
and transforming than he had ever imagined.

Not only is the old reality gone and the new come . . . BUT, the new
that has come is moving quickly to its consummation. The future, God's

Rev. Stephen Pickard is Associate Professor, Head of School of Theology, Charles
Sturt University and Director, St. Mark's National Theological Centre.

[Haworth co-indexing entry note]: "Radical Discipleship for an Ageing Society." Pickard, Stephen.
Co-published simultaneously in *Journal of Religious Gerontology* (The Haworth Pastoral Press, an imprint of
The Haworth Press, Inc.) Vol. 12, No. 3/4, 2001, pp. 181-183; and: *Aging, Spirituality and Pastoral Care: A
Multi-National Perspective* (ed: Elizabeth MacKinlay, James W. Ellor, and Stephen Pickard) The Haworth
Pastoral Press, an imprint of The Haworth Press, Inc., 2001, pp. 181-183. Single or multiple copies of this arti-
cle are available for a fee from The Haworth Document Delivery Service [1-800-342-9678, 9:00 a.m. - 5:00
p.m. (EST). E-mail address: getinfo@haworthpressinc.com].

181

future, is rushing headlong towards the apostle–the whole of this created order. The apostle is overwhelmed at times. Everything is compressed. We live in the end times. "The time is short. . . . the world in its present form is passing away." God's new kingdom and Christ will appear on the scene at any moment. The time of this world is drawing to a rapid close. The Parousia–the final coming of the Messiah–is imminent.

"The time is short." Who says so? The preacher this morning says so. Yet if 1 were honest my imagination is not gripped like Paul by the prospect of an imminent end of the world order, though of course at times it feels frighteningly close. But "the time is short" for me personally. Such is my place in the world; late forties; the horizon of possibilities seem to be expanding not contracting. In fact there are too many tasks, challenges and projects. 1 am overwhelmed with the sheer abundance of possibilities. My fear is simple: I'll run out of time. I'm still in the doing mode not yet into being! Underlying this is a sense of my own mortality. I will die. The present form of my life is passing away; in fact quite quickly.

"The time is short." Who says so? The prophets of our times say so. Time is running out for our environment, the sustainability of our institutions, the Church, ourselves–for we are here for a season and a day. Who amongst us does not feel that the time is short for the late great planet earth?

The time is short and we are confronted with one of those fundamental questions: How shall we live when the time is so short? In our Scripture reading for today the apostle recommends the following: Those who have wives or husbands, they should live as if, in the coming kingdom, a whole new set of relationships will be the order of the day. It is quite simple: those who mourn as if they did not, those who rejoice as if they were not happy. How odd all this seems! How contradictory. Apparently neither tears, not laughter are to be the final determination of our life and being.

But there is more. The apostle also recommends that those who buy something, live as if it were not theirs to keep; those who use the things of the world as if they were not engrossed in them–"have no dealings with them."

This touches a raw nerve in us. We are under the spell of our Western acquisitiveness. We gather, collect, own, hoard, store-up. But is has no permanence. We cannot take it with us and the time is short for our life here so what's the point.

In view of the shortness of time the apostle recommends a radical Christian discipleship. His ethic is one that challenges the idolatries of the age: the family, the indulgent, narcissistic self; the greed of the social economic order. It is the kind of radical discipleship spoken of by the great theologians and practitioners of the faith in our day. I think of Dietrich Bonhoeffer's *Cost of Discipleship* and Kari Barth's reflections on the same topic, or the remarkable life of Mother Teresa.

What about life in an ageing society? This issue of the journal, coming from the conference held in Canberra in January 2000 is about a different paradigm.

It is not "the time is short" but "it's longer than you think!"

We may not overcome our mortality but we will surely succeed in stretching out the term of our natural lives at the 'backend' so to speak. We will have a much longer life at the older end of the life span. How shall we live when the time has expanded rather than shortened?

In particular what does a radical Christian discipleship look like in the ageing society of the coming millennium? How shall we live in a society, as it gets increasingly older? What idolatries do we need to name and depower. For a start we shall need a theology of pastoral care that includes 'nourishing another.' It sounds simple enough but in our cruel times it is in fact a radical option, especially in the context of an ageing people where cries for euthanasia exert such pressure.

What does radical discipleship look like in what is referred to as the 'sandwich years.' Must it mean exhaustion and frustration still caring for the younger generation yet also attending to the more aged? How can joy be embraced in the middle years?

Whether the time is 'short' theologically or longer anthropologically there still remains a call to a radical discipleship. As one person said: "if I had my time over again I would pick more daisies." They meant of course that they would use the time they had to attend to what was nourishing for self and the other. Certainly such a radical discipleship would include learning to travel a little lighter, as if not engrossed in the things we buy, and use. How easy it is to become preoccupied with 'things' and fail to attend to the real needs of self and others. An ageing society brings us up sharply at this point for the frail and older ones around us require nourishing. And it is a mutual nourishing for in our care for them we discover over and over again the source of our own humanity and our neighbours. This is one of the gifts when the time is longer than you think!

The world in its present form is passing away. This is so true. A new world of an ageing society with new challenges is upon us. And the time is short for us to respond with care and grace.

Let us ask for God's grace to begin a new pilgrimage in an ageing world among an ageing people. We travel with the grace and energy of the Saviour who is the same yesterday, today and forever.

Index

Numbers followed by "f" indicate figures; "t" following a page number indicates tabular material.

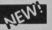